HEAI
&
REVOLUTION

THE NICARAGUAN EXPERIENCE

"God gives health
and the revolution
maintains it."

(A community health worker)

Richard Garfield & Glen Williams

British Library Cataloguing in Publication Data

Garfield, Richard *1953* –
Health and Revolution: the Nicaraguan experience
1. Nicaragua. Health services
I. Title II. Williams, Glen
362.1'097285

ISBN 0 85598 131 8
ISBN 0 85598 132 6 pbk

Published by Oxfam, 274 Banbury Road, Oxford OX2 7DZ.
Designed by Oxfam Design Studio.
Printed by TEK Print Limited.
Typeset in 10 point Times Roman.

Contents

Note: Except where another source is given, the data for the charts in the text are given in full in Appendices 1 to 6. The sources for the data are given in Appendix 7.

Foreword

In publishing this book on health and revolution in Nicaragua, Oxfam hopes to make a major contribution to the public perception of that country. Fundamental changes have taken place in the lives of ordinary Nicaraguans during the ten years since July 1979. In that month the Somoza dictatorship was overthrown by the Sandinistas and Nicaragua has hardly left the headlines of the world press since. However, attention paid by the media has focused more often than not on political and ideological issues with the result that the development experience that was rooted in the Sandinista Revolution has been largely overlooked.

This book is about one of the most fundamental and challenging development policies undertaken following the revolution, namely the attempt to improve the health of a whole nation. Numerous successful health reforms were initiated in the early 1980s, but as time passed and circumstances changed, many difficult choices on health policy faced the Nicaraguan Government and mistakes were inevitably made.

Oxfam has worked in Nicaragua for over twenty years and many of the projects that we have supported have been in the field of primary health care, from the training of traditional birth attendants to mass vaccination campaigns, from the purchase of rainproof clothing and wellington boots for health promoters on the Atlantic Coast to the training of community health workers. We have seen the measurable improvements in health which occurred as a result of the enthusiastic commitment of government and people, and how these improvements have been jeopardised by the deepening economic crisis resulting from the *Contra* war and the political isolation of the country.

We feel that this book tells an important story. At the same time it debunks both the extreme views of Nicaragua as either a socialist utopia or a totalitarian police state. What emerges from its pages are the realities of the lives of ordinary people and an account of how Nicaragua, a Third World country not only beset by problems of poverty, debt and falling prices for its main exports but also by natural disaster and war, has struggled to overcome the obstacles to progress.

The Nicaraguan model of health care delivery can serve other countries facing similar circumstances. Though the decisions on priorities and methods may be different, the debates that need to take place will often be the same. This book will therefore be of interest not just to those concerned with Nicaragua but to all those engaged in constructing sustainable systems that improve the health conditions of the world's poor.

Peter Sollis

Oxford, September 1989

Preface

I first visited Nicaragua in 1980 for what I thought would be a brief visit. From the airport I was whisked off to a seminary where government health leaders were formulating national policy on breastfeeding. By nightfall I seemed to be the only one anxious for the meeting to finish. Such enthusiasm and commitment were hardly characteristic of the health officials I had known in other countries. This hunger for action and results proved to be irresistible. Soon, I found myself part of the system.

I was assigned, in turn, to tasks in the offices of nursing, malaria, epidemiology and the public health school. Over a two-year period I worked as a data analyst, rural administrator, trainer of health volunteers, and public health educator.

My first exposure to rural Nicaragua was with Ania, the 12-year-old daughter of the middle-class family with whom I stayed in Managua. Ania was simple, gracious and yet enormously tough; a year earlier she had killed a member of the Somoza regime's National Guard in the insurrection which brought the Sandinistas to power. When I met her she was in charge of literacy training in a rural community near the small town of Acoyapa, in Chontales province, six hours' drive and a half-hour ride on horseback from Managua. The household where Ania stayed was made of sticks and straw and housed eight people, a pig and two goats. The nearest neighbour lived ten minutes' walk away. These people were just starting to enjoy some of the fruits of the revolution. Their crops brought a better price, they were able to buy a kerosene lamp, and they expected a steady supply of staples like cooking oil, soap and salt. New health posts and schools were being built throughout the province. Like thousands of other adults throughout the country, they were also learning to read and write.

The *Contra* war changed all that. Chontales province has been one of the areas repeatedly attacked by the US-backed *Contra* rebel forces. Since 1984 three clinics in the area have been destroyed, two others damaged in *Contra* attacks and 15 closed due to the war. A team of health experts from Harvard University surveyed health conditions in Acoyapa in 1987[1], and found that a surprising 70% of mothers were still receiving prenatal care. But immunisation coverage had fallen because of the danger of *Contra* attacks on health workers and families: only 40% of the children had immunisation cards that were up to date. More than half of the people had a friend or relative who was killed in the war, and a quarter had been attacked by *Contras* in or near their homes. These attacks had forced many people to abandon subsistence farming and seek safety in the town of Acoyapa or elsewhere. It was a familiar pattern, repeated in many places throughout the country.

The war in Nicaragua has had devastating effects on the whole country, particularly on civilians living in the main war zones. Concern about the effects of United States policies towards Central America was an important factor - but by no means the only factor - in my decision to write about health in Nicaragua.

When I began working in Nicaragua, however, the thought of writing a book about the changes that were taking place in the country's health system was far from my mind. As an active participant in some of those changes, I lacked the time and the detached perspective needed to write about them. Eventually I returned to the United States and in 1985 I joined the Faculty of Medicine at Columbia University in New York. But I continued to visit Nicaragua and to assist the Nicaraguan Ministry of Health (MINSA) in planning, evaluation and training. Gradually, the idea of writing a book about health in Nicaragua formed itself in my mind.

But all too often, I thought, books about health in socialist countries revealed more about the good intentions of the nation's leaders than about the results of their policies. I wanted to write a book that would present a more critical - and therefore more useful - account of the processes of change in Nicaragua's health system during a time of enormous upheaval. For such a book, a wider, more detached perspective was needed.

In Glen Williams I found a co-author who brought such a perspective to the analysis of Nicaragua's experiment in primary health care, and was also able to help tell the 'story' of that experiment in non-technical language. We met soon after he visited Nicaragua to write about the sharp decline in infant mortality during the first few years of the Revolution. By the summer of 1986 we had begun working on the first chapters of this book. We have tried to communicate the freshness, originality and openness of Nicaragua's system, as well as the infectious enthusiasm and commitment of those who have helped to create and shape it. The issues they face will be on the international health agenda for many years to come.

Richard Garfield

1 September 1989

Acknowledgements

Most of the information for this book comes from Nicaraguans who are involved in - and affected by - the rapid changes which have taken place in the country's health care system in the past decade. They include doctors, nurses, midwives, pharmacists, traditional birth attendants, health volunteers, civil servants, nuns and priests, peasants and urban workers, community and political leaders, government policy makers and planners, leaders of non-governmental organisations, as well as mothers, fathers and children. Their importance as sources of information is acknowledged to some extent through direct quotes in the text, but these reflect only a small part of their immense input into the book.

We have also made extensive use of statistical information provided by the Nicaraguan Ministry of Health and other government institutions, the Pan American Health Association, the Inter-American Development Bank, the Latin American Demographic Centre (CELADE) and other research and development institutions. We have also drawn on published and unpublished studies of health and development in Nicaragua and other Latin American countries.

We have been encouraged by Nicaraguan health leaders, especially by Commander Dora Maria Tellez, Leonel Arguello, Carolina Siu, Enrique Morales and Ivan Tercero. Valuable assistance was also provided by Ennio Cufino and Fernando Lezcano of UNICEF, and by Miguel Marquez, Antonio Pages and Isabel Turcios of the Pan American Health Organisation. We are also indebted to David Morley and Leonor Huper for encouragement and support.

OXFAM (UK) and NOVIB provided the financial assistance needed to make this book possible, and the Nicaragua Health Fund also contributed.

Numerous *internacionalistas* have made crucial contributions to the book. Sally McIntyre (USA) co-authored Chapter 8 ('Women's Health'), Fritz Muller of Holland co-authored Chapter 11 ('Medicines and Medical Equipment') and Peter Sollis (UK) co-authored Chapter 13 ('Health in a Survival Economy').

Key material was also provided by Celine Woznica (USA) on community participation in Ciudad Sandino for Chapter 4, by Tim Takaro and Susan Cookson (USA) on the health impact of the *Contra* war for Chapter 6, by Guiseppe Slater (USA) on hospital services for Chapter 7, by Eugenio Taboada (Nicaragua) on the organisation of health services for Chapter 3, by Antonio Dajer (USA) on ambulatory care for Chapter 7, by Jeffrey Gates (USA) on AIDS for Chapter 7, by Ennio Cufino (Italy) on child health programmes for Chapter 9 and by Tom Frieden (USA) on community participation and medical education for Chapters 4 and 11.

Valuable editorial reviews were provided by Alan Meyers, Evelyn Mauss, William Bower, Harris Huberman, Paul Schneider, Tom Frieden, Sarah Jackson, Tim Takaro, Susan Cookson, Antonio Dajer, Jonathan

Fox, Katheryn McGarrity, Antonio Ugalde, Michael Zalkin, Eddy Coyle, Claudia Garcia-Moreno, Peter Sollis and George Davey-Smith. Translations were made by Esperanza Soriano, editorial assistance was provided by Paul Schneider and Robert Gern. Oxfam Publications Department handled the process of production with efficiency and sensitivity.

To all these colleagues, partners and friends, we express our thanks.

Richard Garfield and Glen Williams

New York and Oxford
1 September 1989

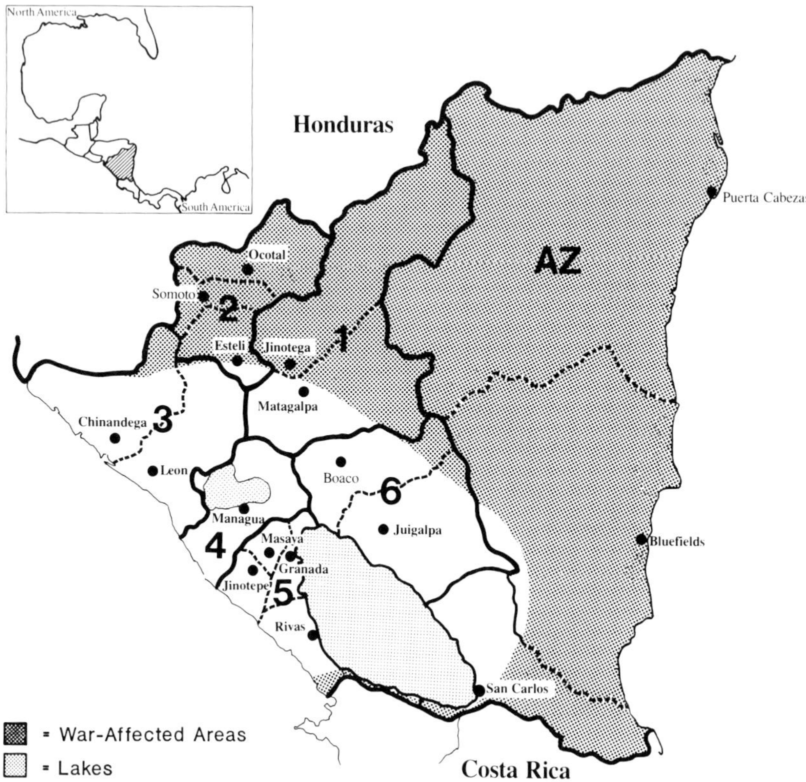

Region	Department	Population*	City
1	Nueva Segovia	114,100	Ocotal
	Madriz	82,800	Somoto
	Esteli	150,500	Esteli
2	Chinandega	311,100	Chinandega
	Leon	327,000	Leon
3	Managua	965,800	Managua
4	Masaya	226,800	Masaya
	Carazo	166,000	Jinotepe
	Grenada	132,600	Granada
	Rivas	139,500	Rivas
5	Chontales	116,400	Juigalpa
	Boaco	105,700	Boaco
6	Matagalpa	353,200	Matagalpa
	Jinotega	100,600	Jinotega
AZ#	North Zelaya	95,000	Puerta Cabezas
	South Zelaya	171,300	Bluefields
	Rio San Juan	53,300	San Carlos

*Estimated Population in 1988 (Source: INEC)

#AZ is the Autonomous Zone

Chapter 1: Introduction

EL NUEVO DIARIO

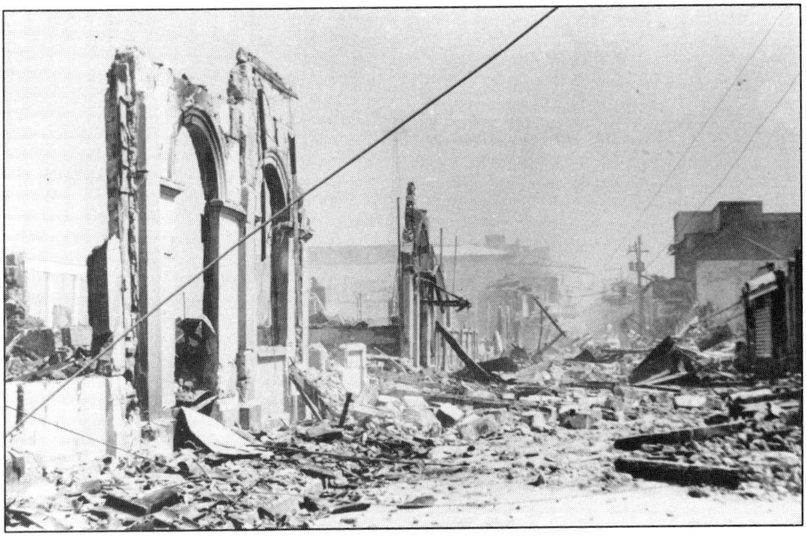

Street scene, Managua, after the earthquake in 1972.

At one minute past midnight on 23 December 1972 a massive earthquake hit the Nicaraguan capital, Managua. It killed 10,000 people, injured 20,000 more, and left three quarters of the city's 400,000 residents homeless.[1] Panic reigned. Survivors rushed the injured to El Retiro — the city's central hospital — only to find it in ruins. Few doctors or nurses were on hand in any case. Many were busy caring for injured members of their own families or protecting the rubble of their homes from thieves. Others, fearing the deluge of patients at the hospital, simply stayed away.

The rule of the jungle quickly became the norm. Those who gained most were, as usual, President Anastasio Somoza Debayle and his associates. They went into action immediately, speculating in land and pocketing millions of dollars in aid, food and supplies intended for earthquake victims.

The most visible aid from the Government of the United States was barbed wire. It was used to cordon off the central city business district, supposedly to discourage looters. In fact, the barbed wire made looting easier for Somoza's armed forces. The US Government and voluntary agencies also sent large quantities of food and medical supplies, but little of this aid reached those in need.

A US mobile military hospital, with a full contingent of surgical and support staff, arrived within 48 hours of the earthquake. The surgical unit was set up within the confines of the US embassy, where patients with the right connections were admitted for treatment. So few were treated that doctors and nurses passed their time by playing volleyball in the embassy compound. Meanwhile, outside the embassy gate, thousands of people with serious injuries waited in vain for treatment. It was a scene which aptly symbolised Nicaraguan society: a poor majority were excluded by a tiny elite sustained by the United States.

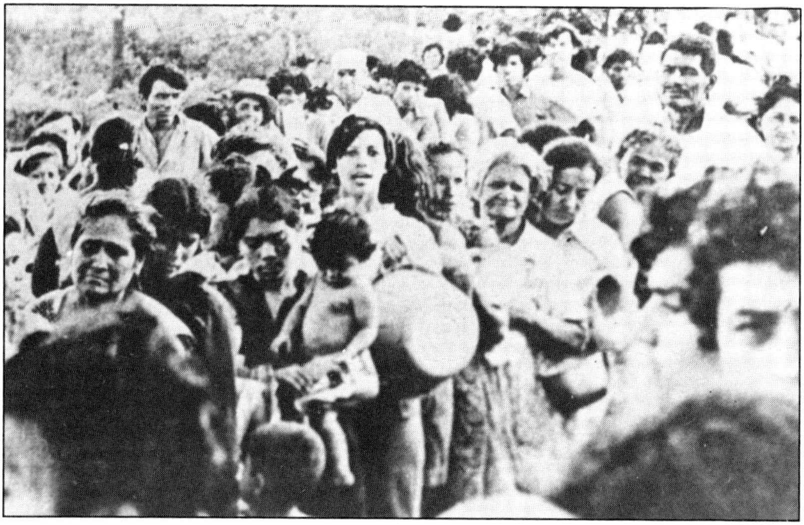

EL NUEVO DIARIO

People made homeless by the 1972 earthquake queue for emergency food rations. Millions of dollars' worth of aid were misappropriated by President Somoza and his associates.

Among the economic links between the two countries was the infamous 'Plasmaferesis' laboratory in Managua. Arnoldo Ramos was a Cuban expatriate who found safe haven in Nicaragua after the failed 'Bay of Pigs' invasion of Cuba in 1961. He ran a profitable pharmaceutical company in partnership with the Somoza family. In an ingenious new scheme, Ramos and Somoza began exporting blood plasma to the United States. The 'Plasmaferesis' laboratory quickly became one of Managua's major industries, employing 500 workers and producing 15% of the world's supply of blood plasma.

By 1975, thousands of people earned a living selling their blood for $5 a pint to the laboratory. The plasma was then sold for about $30 to dealers in the US. Since blood donors also received a meal, 'vampire Ramos' (as he was known) was never short of would-be donors. Many had recently come to the city from the rural north, where the Somozas had seized their lands for tobacco, sugar, and cotton plantations. The poor districts of Managua overflowed with thousands of displaced ex-peasant farmers who survived by selling blood during most of the year and harvesting export crops on plantations for a couple of months.

The plasma business eventually contributed to the downfall of the Somoza regime. In 1977, the newspaper *La Prensa* reported horrific abuses occurring in the 'Plasmaferesis' laboratory. Front page photos showing cadavers wholly drained of blood provoked a storm of public anger. The Somoza regime's response was to kill Pedro Joaquin Chamorro, editor of *La Prensa*, on 10 January 1978. A massive public reaction followed immediately. Angry crowds invaded the hospital where Chamorro's body was being held, and 40,000 people accompanied his coffin to the cemetery. Defying the much-feared National Guard, protesters put Somoza-owned businesses to the torch. Along with banks, factories and finance houses, the infamous 'Plasmaferesis' laboratory went up in flames.

This burst of outrage was the spark from which the Sandinista National Liberation Front (FSLN) organised a general insurrection and, 18 months later, overthrew the dictatorship. Somoza fought fiercely to maintain power. About 35,000* people died in the revolutionary war and much of the country's economic and social infrastructure was reduced to ruins.[2] When the Sandinistas finally took power on 19 July 1979, they inherited the highest per capita foreign debt in Latin America. The revolutionary Government faced the immense task of reconstructing a bankrupt nation which for more than four decades had suffered under one of Latin America's most brutal, corrupt dictatorships.

The Sandinistas

Formed in 1961, the FSLN developed a philosophy consisting of a mix of Marxism, radical Christianity and nationalism. The Front took its name from the national hero Augusto Cesar Sandino, a revolutionary general whose guerrilla troops fought an occupying force of US marines to a standstill between 1927 and 1933. A thorn in the side of the US-backed Nicaraguan Government of the day, Sandino was murdered in 1934 on the orders of Anastasio Somoza Garcia, then head of the National Guard. In 1936 Somoza assumed the Presidency, starting a dynasty which lasted 43 years.[3]

The FSLN proclaimed its intention of establishing a state based on three guiding principles: political pluralism, a mixed economy, and non-alignment in international affairs. They would form a government dedicated to pursuing 'the logic of the majority' by promoting the interests of the poor and marginalised — those who had suffered most under the Somoza regime.[4]

*** Estimates of deaths vary — some sources put the numbers of deaths as high as 50,000.**

Primary Health Care

A central plank in the FSLN's political platform was a revolution in health and social welfare. Upon coming to power, the new Government boosted health spending to make it the second largest item (after education) in the state budget.[5] A massive programme was begun to make health care available throughout the country. Thousands of health workers were trained and sent to rural areas. Community volunteers were recruited and local health councils were established to implement campaigns promoting childhood immunisation, malaria control and environmental hygiene.

These efforts rode a wave of international interest in primary health care. The new primary health care strategy, proclaimed by the World Health Organisation in 1978, concentrated on simple, inexpensive health technologies.[6] (See also Chapter 3.) The aim was to improve the health of the whole population by concentrating on disease prevention, health education in nutrition and hygiene, the provision of safe water and basic sanitation, universal access to basic curative services, maternal and child care and immunisation against common diseases.

Nicaraguans

Ten years after the FSLN came to power, here is what some Nicaraguans think of their health system:

Maria Lourdes Espinoza and her husband Jose have a small farm near the town of Jalapa, about ten kilometres from the border with Honduras. Their house is made of rough timber and tin sheets. A pig sits in the doorway and smoke from the kitchen seeps through a gap in the wall. They grow corn, keep a few chickens and have some mango and grapefruit trees. The oldest of their six children is nine, the youngest two, and Maria is now six months pregnant. How has the revolution affected her health and that of her family?

"Life here is still very hard, but at least we don't have to worry much about getting medicines any more. The Government has built a clinic and a feeding centre for children in town. It doesn't matter if you have money or not. They treat you fairly and they treat you well, like you really deserve it. How many of my children would still be alive if they didn't care about us at the health centre? This Government doesn't have much, but they do as much with it as possible."

Lorenzo Olivares, once a member of a cooperative near Ocotal, now lives with his three children in a settlement for families displaced by the war 30 miles south of the Honduran border. At one time he was an enthusiastic supporter of the revolution. He became a health volunteer in 1981 and took part in the mass campaigns against malaria, dengue, polio and measles. In 1986 anti-government rebels (*Contras*) attacked his cooperative with mortars, grenades and machine guns, killing three adults and two children, including Lorenzo's wife and youngest child. The settlement where he now lives is safer but the nearest health post is ten miles away. Bitter and disillusioned, he feels that the revolution's slogans are a mockery:

"We had great plans and hopes, but what can I do now? A government official said they would give us a new clinic, but for six months we've been waiting and there are a lot of sick people here. They say the Sandinista revolution means health, but all I've seen is death."

Leonel Arguello finished his medical studies in 1980 and was posted to a remote part of the Atlantic Coast for 12 months. It was a rude awakening for a young doctor from the capital city:

"I come from a family with a social conscience, who supported the revolution. But until I worked in a really isolated area I didn't understand what the revolution meant. I worked among people who had never heard of a doctor, had never tasted sugar, and had never seen ice. But what made the biggest impression on me was the serenity with which the *campesinos* accepted the deaths of their children. Even the most destitute parents in Managua would cry if their child died. The *campesinos* didn't. Their faces showed stony acceptance. Their lives had never been anything more than misery, anyhow. It took the revolution to open their eyes to other possibilities."

Teresa Martinez Cruz has helped hundreds of mothers bring their babies into the world during the past 28 years. She has never been to school and can barely read or write. In 1982 she attended a part-time training course run by the Ministry of Health for traditional birth attendants. Today, she is the health organiser in her community, the satellite town of Ciudad Sandino about ten kilometres outside Managua. For Teresa, the revolution has meant recognition:

"In the old days, the doctors and nurses wouldn't even talk with us. Now I work as a member of the health team for this community. It's nice to have that official support. But what's even more important is that my neighbours appreciate my work and know they can depend on me."

Julio Zaragosa has a flourishing pharmacy in the working class neighbourhood of San Judas in Managua. He owns a car and lives in a comfortable home in the affluent suburb of Bolonia. His two sons attend boarding school in the USA. For Julio the revolution spells nothing but disaster:

"Health care was bad before and it's just as bad now. Before, only the rich had good health care. The poor lined up for charity, and the middle class went to private doctors. Now it seems that no-one can afford a doctor, so more people go to the public hospitals and clinics, which are always full and filthy. The Government says there is more medical care now. Where is it? There must be some little old lady somewhere getting it all because I can't see it anywhere. This dictatorship is worse than Somoza's. They've given all our products to Russia and attack those of us who try to earn a living. The country is being ruined."

Dora Osorio is a mother of five and works as a domestic servant in Managua. Deserted by her husband three years ago, she struggles hard to make ends meet. For Dora, the revolution meant she could give birth in hospital and her children could receive free health care. But recently things have changed:

"I know the hospitals because I go there when it's time to have a baby. It's pretty good there, but you only go to hospital when you really have to. Before the revolution you had to pay for health care. I only took my children to the doctor if they were really ill. Then came the revolution and they made the public clinics much better and you didn't have to pay. We used to go there a lot. But now you have to pay for the medicines, and I can't afford it any more. I know our Government is doing the best it can, but I wish it would do better."

Don Chema, an itinerant cobbler, lives in El Crucero, a wind-swept crossroads 30 kilometres south of Managua. For him, the revolution means that the Government finally gives importance to the poor:

"Before the revolution, nuns used to provide some health care. But it's only since 1979 that the Government has done anything. Now you can go to the clinic in the morning, and you can be sure they will treat you the same day. They treat you with respect and don't ask how much money you have. There are even some doctors there from Holland or Germany. You see, people care about our poor little country now."

The Country

Wedged between Honduras in the north and Costa Rica in the south, Nicaragua is the largest of the six countries of the Central American isthmus. The population is growing rapidly (see Figure 1.1).

The country has three main geographic regions. On the western coast are fertile plains which are home to 60% of the people. Volcanic activity has left a fertile soil and the two great lakes, Lake Managua and Lake Nicaragua. The central uplands are a chain of rugged hills and mountains which run from the northern border almost down to Costa Rica in the south. This region has a temperate climate but is short of water, and is more sparsely populated. On the east is the so-called Atlantic Coast — something of a misnomer for a region of rain forests, savannah, swamps and lagoons. It occupies almost half the national territory but has only 10% of the population.

The country is dotted with towns, villages, and dispersed rural

Fig. 1.1

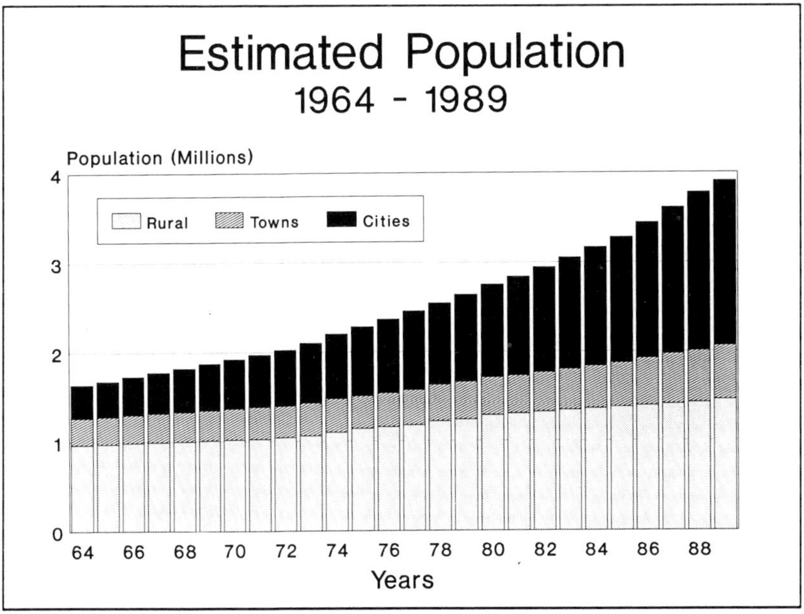

From 1979 to 1989, the estimated national population rose by 48%. Most of this rise was in cities (more than 20,000 inhabitants), whose population grew by 74% during this period. In rural areas (less than 5,000 inhabitants), the population is believed to have grown by only 27%. The country's population has doubled since 1971.

dwellings.[7] More than 5,000 communities are located in 135 municipalities. The traditional geopolitical division is the department, of which there are 16. To encourage decentralisation the departments were organised in 1982 into regions.[8] The Pacific and upland zones are now divided into six regions. Since 1988 the two departments on the Atlantic coast have been designated the 'autonomous zone' and enjoy a high measure of local self-government (see map facing page 1).

The Pacific and upland regions, first colonised by Spain in the early sixteenth century, are ethnically and culturally homogeneous. Almost all the people are Mestizo (of mixed Spanish and indigenous Indian ancestry), Spanish-speaking, and Roman Catholic. The Atlantic Coast, a sphere of British influence for more than two centuries, is home to six different ethnic groups. Half the population consists of Spanish-speaking Mestizos who have migrated from the Pacific region. The largest ethnic minority is the Miskito people, descendants of indigenous Indians and Afro-Caribbean slaves or immigrants. The Miskitos still speak their own language and live mainly in the north. The five non-Mestizo minorities of the Atlantic Coast, the largest of which are English-speaking Creoles, belong mostly to the Moravian or other Protestant churches.

The economies of the three regions are quite distinct. The Pacific region produces cotton and sugar for export as well as maize, rice and beans for domestic consumption. The central uplands are used primarily for cattle raising and coffee production. On the Atlantic Coast, where communications are poorly developed and transport is mainly by river or dirt road, the main economic activities are lumbering, gold mining, fishing and subsistence agriculture.

Before the revolution a small group of landowners and entrepreneurs, headed by the Somoza family, controlled the economy of the Pacific region. Thousands of small-scale farmers, forced off their land on the coastal plain to make way for export crops, worked as itinerant seasonal labourers on large estates. Wealth and income were highly skewed. The average per capita income of the richest 5% of the population was $5,409.[9] This was 25 times that of the poorest 50% of the people, whose income averaged less than $300 a year in the late 1970s. Annual per capita rural incomes varied from $90 to $225 by region. The Somoza family alone controlled a quarter of the country's agricultural land as well as the national airline, a bank, the two television stations, a pharmaceutical firm, and more than 40 of the country's largest companies. The economy of the Pacific region was closely linked to the United States, which bought most of its exports and supplied almost all its imports.

The Somozas had little direct involvement in the economy of the Atlantic Coast. Communications between the two sides of the country were almost non-existent. There were no roads, railways or telephone links between the Atlantic Coast and Managua. The exploitation of the region's forests, fisheries and mineral resources was left largely to US-based multinational companies. As one Miskito leader remarked: "Somoza may have neglected us, but at least he left us alone."

Despite its agricultural economy, Nicaragua is one of the most highly urbanised countries in Latin America[10] (see Figure 1.2). About a million people are believed to live in Managua, whose population has more than doubled since the earthquake of 1972.[11] About a million more live in other cities and towns, while another million live in villages and rural areas.

About this book

This book tells the stories of farmers and artisans, doctors and nurses, folk healers and community volunteers. It analyses how the dramatic changes in health care introduced by the Sandinistas affect them. It describes monumental efforts to make health care available to the poor majority through a new system of primary health care.

Perhaps the most important component of the primary care strategy

Fig. 1.2

Basic Data, 1988

Population	3.6 Million
Infant Mortality Rate	68 per 1000 Live Births
Under-5-Year-Old Mortality Rate	100 per 1000 Population
Crude Birth Rate	42 per 1000 Population
Crude Death Rate	9 per 1000 Population
Population Growth Rate	3.4% per Year
Life Expectancy at Birth	63 Years
Percent of Population Rural	43%
Total Average Births per Woman	5.8

Sources: UNICEF, *Datos basicos e indicadores economicos, humanos, politicos, y sociales sobre Nicaragua*, Managua: UNICEF, 1988.
UNICEF: *Statistics on children in UNICEF assisted countries*, New York: UNICEF: 1987.

outlined by the World Health Organisation in 1978 was 'political will'. This is probably the only element of the Nicaraguan system to be unchanged throughout the 1980s. The Sandinistas began with lofty goals and costly assumptions about what good health care would require. Dialogue among health professionals and demands from the population have subsequently led to more modest approaches. Five years of economic strangulation and eight years of war have dictated a low-cost, more sustainable approach. This change has involved revisions in the number and type of health professionals trained, the number and type of medicines distributed, the nature of health campaigns, the role of international assistance and the type of medical care practised.

The book examines efforts to involve communities in setting priorities and implementing health programmes. The weaknesses, limitations, and failures of the new health system are analysed, as well as its achievements. This is not a story of overnight miracles, but of hard-won successes, daunting challenges and painful failures. Progress has not been simple or easy. It has emerged through a process of grappling with poverty, ignorance, poor management, simplistic idealism, opposition from doctors, public apathy and corruption.

Despite a decade of natural disasters, political upheaval, economic decline, and war, Nicaragua has developed and maintained a system of primary health care which responds to the needs of most people. This system continues to grow and evolve despite overwhelming limitations. The book examines how this has occurred and what it means for other poor nations wishing to extend the reach of their health services. There are lessons here for other societies where economic decline and deteriorating health systems seem to have become permanent.

Chapters 2 to 7 chronicle the evolution of health services during the past decade. Chapters 8 to 13 analyse topics of particular interest in more detail. Key topics are highlighted at the end of each chapter and discussed in more depth in Chapter 14. Pertinent data are presented in tables and graphs near the text where they are discussed. Data for the figures as well as additional health-related data and bibliographic references are presented in appendices.

Chapter 2: From Chaos to Crisis: Prior to 1979

"In Nicaragua life is a slow death. I can't live it, nobody can. I'm going to fight for life in Nicaragua."
(Dr. Oscar Danilo Rosales, killed in action, 27 August 1967)

Many doctors made a good living under Somoza. Some, especially leading members of the *Colegio de Medicos* and Ministry of Health officials, were vociferous supporters of the regime. Many others made a stand against the system. One of the first was Oscar Danilo Rosales, a highly respected young pathologist. In July 1967 he resigned his post as Director of the Department of Pathology at the Medical School in Leon to join the Sandinista guerrillas. In his letter of resignation to the Rector of the University[1] he explained:[2]

"In view of the current political situation in Nicaragua... I believe that it is the responsibility of all intellectuals...to join the ranks of the army of Nicaragua, according to the ideals of the immortal Sandino and under the flag of the FSLN."

A month later, he wrote what was to be his last letter from a mountain hide-out: "Tomorrow everything will be different. New airs will be breathed in our country, an aura of justice will prevail and we'll end hunger and misery, malnutrition, ill-health, illiteracy, and lack of liberty, from which our people suffer."

On 27 August 1967, in one of the first battles between the FSLN and the National Guard, Rosales and several other guerrillas were killed in an aerial napalm attack. Twelve years later, the new Sandinista-led Government renamed the Leon Medical School in his memory.

Alejandro Davila Bolanos was another early medical revolutionary. Bolanos was a physician, naturalist, anthropologist, literary critic, linguist and poet. He made a life-long study of the history, languages and medicines of the indigenous peoples of Central America. He also collected 3,000 texts on these subjects while he worked with peasants and their organisations in the north of the country, (see Box). A respected society figure in Esteli., his home was a hub of local literary and political activity.[3]

Pamphlets that Bolanos published in the 1960s for peasant farmers showed a great understanding of the conditions of deprivation in which they lived:

"Good food, housing, money and employment contribute to maintaining health... If your boss doesn't give you meat, demand it or ask for eggs in its place... Give your children all the milk they want... A garden, however small it may be, is better than a doctor... If you have a well, cover the top... Struggle to improve your salary... When the children are sick give them boiled water... Bathe daily with soap, including the private parts... Improve your house by separating the sleeping and cooking areas and putting in big windows. Separate the place for animals from the food storage area. Send your children to the nearest school and keep yourself informed of their progress. Get together with other *campesino* men like yourself and discuss how to improve the school. Alcohol will make you poorer, more unhappy, and a disgrace. If you are an honourable man, marry the woman with whom you live... When your woman or children are ill, care for them. Don't spend your money on witchcraft or false cures. A pregnant woman needs more milk, vegetables and meat than normal. If your woman has more than two days of pain in labour and still has not given birth, take her to a hospital. If there are a lot of mosquitoes where you live, sleep under mosquito nets. Demand better roads and communications from the government. Don't sell the land where you live, as you must depend on it for your livelihood."

Bolanos worked closely with the Sandinistas. When a general strike broke out in August 1978 in Esteli, he and seven other leaders were arrested and brutally tortured by the National Guard.[4] His precious library was destroyed as 'subversive'.

Released after three months, Bolanos was back at work in Esteli hospital when the final insurrection began in April 1979. He was one of several doctors who stayed in the hospital night and day to treat the injured as Somoza's planes bombed the city. The National Guard stormed the hospital, seized Bolanos, tortured and killed him, and burned his body in front of the hospital. Only three months later, the National Guard was defeated and the revolution for which he gave his life became a reality.

Health status

When the Sandinistas came to power in July 1979, health status in Nicaragua ranked alongside that in Honduras and Bolivia as the worst in continental Latin America. Average life expectancy at birth was estimated at 53 years.[5] This low life expectancy was mainly a result of deaths in the first year of life. One in every eight babies died before reaching one year of age. The main causes were diarrhoeal disease, pneumonia, tetanus, measles and whooping cough. Malnutrition affected more than half of all children. Polio epidemics occurred every few years, leaving hundreds of children permanently disabled.[6]

Some of these problems were beyond the reach of doctors, nurses and midwives. Their roots were social and economic — poverty, landlessness, inadequate food supplies, illiteracy, poor housing and sanitation, and lack of clean drinking water.[7]

Yet the health services themselves also bore much of the blame. The country's health system was extremely inefficient and inequitable. Paradoxically, lack of money was not the main problem. The system was relatively well-endowed with funds (including foreign aid), as well as doctors and hospital beds. But the system was severely imbalanced. There were close to 5,000 beds in about 40 hospitals, but there were less than 200 health centres in the entire country.[8] Some of these health centres were well designed and lavishly equipped, but most operated at under 50% of capacity. The system was riddled with corruption and geared almost exclusively to the needs of the affluent.

It was estimated that 90% of Nicaragua's health resources during the 1970s were directed to a mere 10% of the population.[9] Most of the affluent or medically insured lived in Managua and the second-largest city, Leon. They controlled most of the country's land, commerce and industry, and consumed mosdt of the health resources. Among these groups child deaths were about as rare, and life expectancy almost as high, as in North America.

Administrative chaos

Prior to the 1979 revolution Nicaragua's health system was profoundly fragmented. Four separate national institutions and 19 semi-autonomous local agencies were responsible for health services. Because each institution and agency functioned independently, chaos was the norm, with salaries, record-keeping and working practices differing from one town to the next.

The most powerful health institution was not the Ministry of Health, but the National Social Security Institute (INSS), which provided curative health care to salaried employees. With its own hospitals and clinics in Managua and Leon, the INSS controlled half of all health expenditure but provided services to only 8.4% of the population.[10] Health expenditure per person was more than ten times greater for the insured than the uninsured. In 1977, insured patients had more than eight times as many outpatient visits and prescriptions dispensed as the rest of the population. The National Guard also ran its own hospitals and clinics, providing high quality care to soldiers and their relatives.

The Ministry of Health, although responsible for preventive care throughout the country and curative services in rural areas, controlled only 16% of health expenditure — and 75% of this was spent in Managua.[11] Private insurance groups, charitable organisations and local health agencies accounted for most of the remaining health expenditure.

Only 28% of the Nicaraguan population had effective access to any modern health services. An estimated 60% of all health resources were concentrated in Managua, where 25% of the population lived.[12] Other people, especially those in rural areas, remained dependent on traditional healers (*curanderos*) and birth attendants (*parteras*) for health advice and treatment. They might see a doctor only if they went to sell their blood to the 'Plasmaferesis' laboratory in Managua. Whatever public health care did exist under Somoza was curative, except for malaria control. Alta Hooker, a nurse from the Atlantic Coast, recalls conditions before the revolution:

"People were afraid to come to the hospital because they would have to pay. When symptoms started, they took home remedies. By the time they realised they needed help, it was often too late, because they would have to travel for days to reach the hospital. Patients used to appear at the

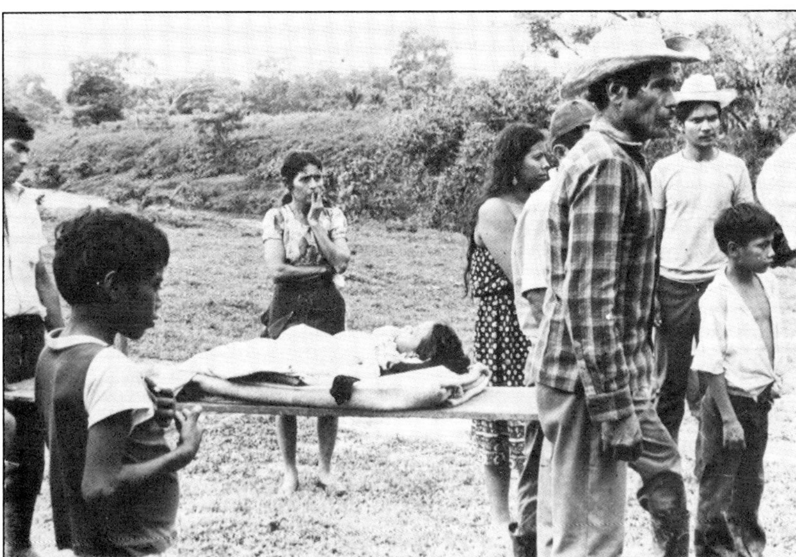

LA PRENSA

A sick child, carried on a home-made stretcher. People sometimes had to walk for days to reach a hospital.

hospital on a home-made stretcher, with a blood pressure of 40. This meant shock, deep shock. I remember one patient who had a ruptured appendix for ten days — that's how long it took them to reach us."

For landless labourers working on privately owned farms and plantations, health care was virtually non-existent. Luis Mendoza, who now works on a state farm, remembers:

"Before the revolution there was no place to go if somebody got sick. We just tried whatever we heard would work. A doctor would have been better of course, but how? The boss paid a doctor to care for his animals, but for us? Why should he? He could always find more workers if we died."

Polio vaccination 'campaigns' were carried out only after epidemics. Such campaigns received the patronage of First Lady Hope Somoza, but their function was essentially symbolic. They were 'too little, too late' to have any impact on transmission of the disease.

Curative care was dispensed largely on an 'ability to pay' basis. In Esteli hospital, for example, a three-tiered system existed. Those who paid a small fee were admitted to large, open wards and received irregular attention. Those who could pay more went to semi-private rooms and were visited daily. Those who could pay well had private rooms and round-the-clock medical attention. Dr. Fernando Silva, now Director of the 'La Mascota' Children's Hospital in Managua, remembers:

"There was care available to the poor, but there was never much and it was of very poor quality. It had all the limitations of charity care — bad doctors, worse medicine, and lack of consideration. Treatment at health centres was even worse. There was always a heap of people waiting around. When the doctor arrived he would begin writing and handing out prescriptions, one after the other. All that mattered was that people got a prescription."

Foreign aid

To alleviate this suffering, many foreign organisations set up hospitals and clinics. Health and development aid from the United States increased sharply after President Kennedy set up the Alliance for Progress in the early 1960s.[13] Many donors were religious and other non-governmental organisations. The biggest donor, however, was the United States Agency for International Development (USAID). Loans and grants from USAID were used to build rural health centres, set up a mobile rural health programme, train doctors, build hospitals, stimulate community participation and improve sanitation. Despite financial incentives and technical assistance, the anarchic, paternalistic, and profit-oriented nature of the Nicaraguan health system defeated USAID's reform efforts. A USAID evaluation in the mid-1970s found:

"... a combination of poor physical plant, lack of equipment, uncleanliness, and poor quality medical attention. No provisions were made to provide these [health] centres, once built, with adequate personnel, supplies, and management support. ... The average health centre operated at about 40% capacity in terms of patient visits per medical hour..." [14]

The major stumbling block to reform was the political and economic system of the country. The evaluation summed up, in a cautious understatement, the effects of the Somoza dictatorship on the health system:

"The long history of one party rule in the country...resulted in a centralised decision-making process with limited delegation of responsibility and authority, which often required the President to personally intervene in issues affecting even small amounts of sector resources. Thus the health sector and many health sector personnel lacked the motivation and innovative-experimental approach necessary to make a major impact on the enormous health problems facing the health agencies..." [15]

Private aid was sometimes more effective. The Evangelical Committee for Aid and Development (CEPAD) was set up by the Protestant Church after the 1972 earthquake in order to bypass the Government in channelling development assistance to rural areas.

CEPAD established and still runs more than 20 clinics in isolated rural communities. Their focus on home gardens, latrines, water systems, breastfeeding and health education has been exemplary.

USAID and other international donors tried to encourage reform within the Government. The major result of this effort was a 1977 meeting of health leaders in Chinandega which developed a blueprint for reform. Plans were made for unifying the various public health agencies into one ministry, coordinating the care provided by hospitals, building more clinics and improving their utilisation, and starting a variety of rural health programmes.

Such reforms, however, threatened powerful leaders and might have undermined the Somoza system of control. None of the major urban programmes called for in Chinandega were ever initiated. Rural programmes begun because of the Chinandega initiative were wholly supported by foreign funds and were subverted to help defend the dictatorship against growing support for the Sandinistas among peasants. In short, as long as the Somoza dynasty remained in power, efforts toward reform of the health system were condemned to failure.

Somoza bombs hospitals

Health workers were considered potential subversives by the Somoza regime because they dealt with a popular concern which the Government ignored. The Government carefully limited the number of doctors and nurses to be trained. FETSALUD, the health workers' union formed in 1974, organised several strikes in hospitals to oppose Somoza. By 1977,

FETSALUD was one of the largest and most important trade unions in the country. The National Guard was reluctant to attack hospital workers with the same fury with which it destroyed other trade unions. The very doctors and nurses they might shoot today could well be needed to care for their own families tomorrow.

In August 1978 FETSALUD led a hunger strike against the dictatorship.[16] As Somoza's position weakened, so did his restraint. Union leaders were jailed, murdered or simply 'disappeared'. Many health workers, especially nurses, left the country because of political harassment or lockouts. Finally, the Guard turned its fury on the hospitals themselves. During the last months of the war four of the country's public hospitals were destroyed and five others were damaged in air or artillery attacks by Somoza Government forces.[17]

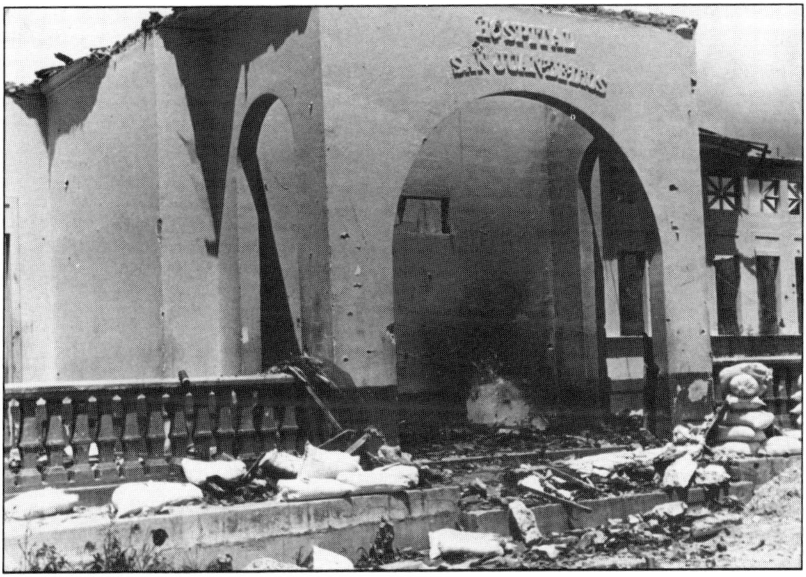

G TELLEZ / NICARAGUA HEALTH FUND

The hospital in Esteli, badly damaged in an air raid by Somoza Government forces towards the end of the insurrection in 1979.

The Sandinistas organise

Meanwhile, growing numbers of doctors, nurses and medical students abandoned hospitals, private practices and universities to join the Sandinista guerrillas. For years, doctors had secretly treated wounded FSLN combatants. Clandestine networks were established to move injured or ill guerrillas out of the country for treatment. Doctors and nurses (including 21 doctors from Germany, Costa Rica, Honduras and Mexico) also trained medical orderlies who were attached to Sandinista combat units. In neighbourhoods of Leon, Esteli and Managua, where the National Guard had already lost effective control, the FSLN established clandestine hospitals where doctors operated on the war-wounded. Many health workers lived a dual life — an official one working in a government hospital or clinic and a secret one treating FSLN guerrillas and their families. It was a perilous existence. Dr. Fernando Silva worked with the FSLN in Managua:

"We would collect needles, syringes, penicillin, gauze, and other medical supplies to send to the countryside and the fighters. I remember the day when the Medical Director came to the Social Security clinic where I was working. He said he was convinced I was working for those sons-of-bitches the Sandinistas. This shook me because my white jacket was bulging with a pistol. I was in the habit of travelling armed because I was treating guerrillas. 'After you finish with these patients, come to my office so that we can talk,' he said. I didn't know what to do. I needed to get rid of the gun. I was trembling with fear that I would be shot because of the gun. There was a man nearby, holding a baby in his arms covered by a blanket. He touched me. 'Don't worry,' he said. He took the gun and put it under the blanket. I was saved from certain death. That night they attacked my house, but I had already fled."

Growing numbers of health professionals became deeply involved in the revolution. Medical students were recruited to treat wounded guerrilla fighters in the mountains. Physicians went 'underground' in the cities to coordinate protests. The current Minister of Health, Dora Maria Tellez, lived both lives:

"To go underground in the city was always very hard. At times there were *companeros* who spent months shut inside a single room. Life in the mountains was physically very hard, but there was the advantage of being together with others."

In the mountains, Sandinistas encountered health problems for which they were wholly unprepared. Omar Cabezas, a guerrilla fighter, noticed white dots which soon grew into ulcers on his legs:

"...around the white dot it was red, red, red ... I figured they would give me a shot to knock it out, because they had a fair supply of medicine [at camp] ... It took three people for my treatment. A *companero* would cut a couple of branches. They put one in each of my hands and another in my mouth so I wouldn't yell ... The gauze came out all covered with pus and blood and chunks of flesh ... Poor Flavio was always in his hammock, depressed because he couldn't figure out what it was. One afternoon he came running up: 'It's leishmaniasis*, leishmaniasis!' like somebody crying out, 'Land, land!' 'What's leishmaniasis?' 'Brother, it's what you've got. It's mountain leprosy, that's leishmaniasis,' he announced."[18]

*** Leishmaniasis is a disease of the skin and mucous membranes caused by a parasitic protozoan.**

By early 1979 activity at the government health facilities, which had been woefully inadequate under normal conditions, ground to a halt. Elizabeth Perez Ode was working as a physician that year in Muy Muy, Matagalpa:

"We had to close the clinic because of the war. All the people were afraid to come out. All we could do was register the dead after the National Guard had finished 'interrogating' suspects."

Hospitals ran out of supplies and had to turn away patients. Many doctors and nurses, fearing attacks by the National Guard, simply stopped reporting for work at hospitals and health centres. In government-held areas, only the Red Cross was able to provide emergency relief — and then only sporadically.[19] The National Guard often prevented the Red Cross from assisting the civilian population, and murdered several Red Cross workers who defied their orders.

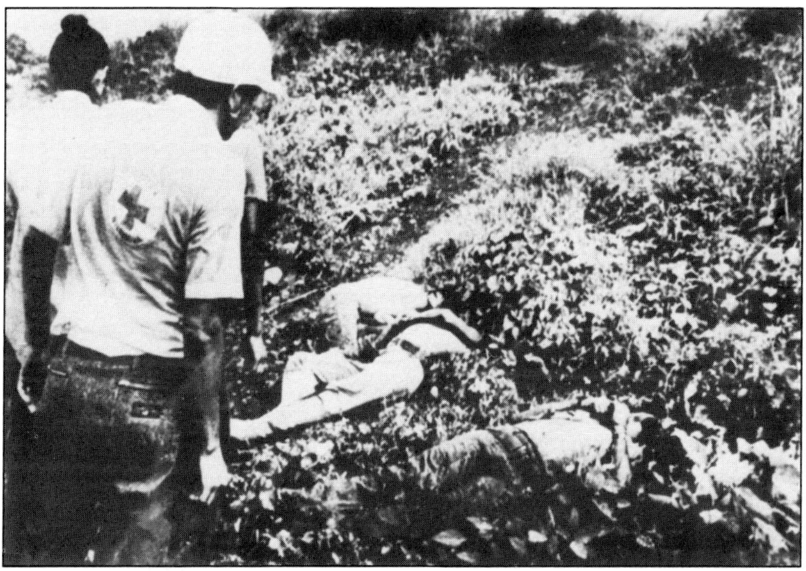

EL NUEVO DIARIO

A site in Managua where the National Guard dumped the bodies of their torture victims, 1979.

In neighbourhoods supporting the Sandinistas, food, water, and other basic supplies ran out as the Government attempted to starve the people into submission. The FSLN responded by organising Civil Defence Committees which acted as provisional local governments, storing and distributing food, water and essential commodities such as kerosene and cooking oil. The Committees also threw up street barricades, deployed lookouts and messengers to support the guerrilla fighters, coordinated health volunteers, trained orderlies to treat the sick and wounded, and

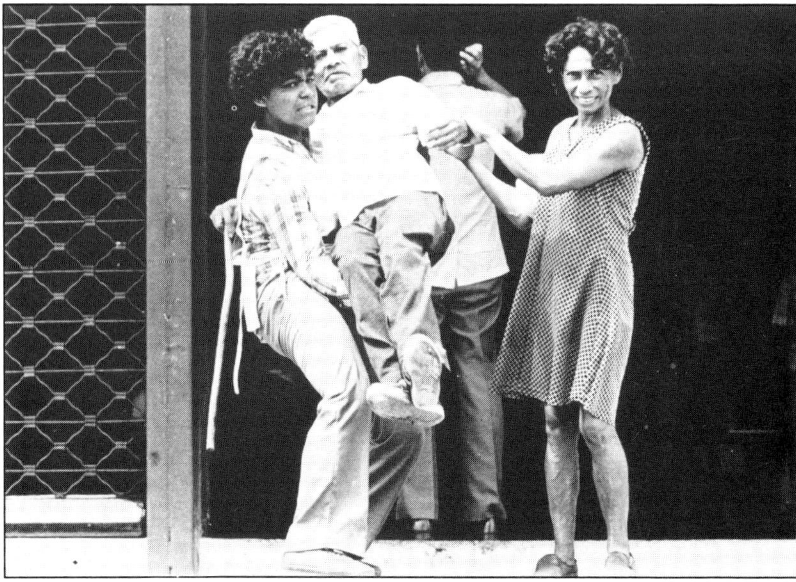

EL NUEVO DIARIO

Red Cross personnel help a patient during the insurrection in 1979. The FSLN set up Civil Defence Committees in many urban areas which took responsibility for medical care and food distribution.

organised the burial of the dead and the disposal of household refuse.

In effect, the National Guard obliged the Sandinistas to create a cadre of dedicated volunteers working in 'liberated' communities.[20] By July 1979, when more than four decades of Somoza rule finally came to an end, the Sandinistas had already established the framework for a system of widespread community decision-making and action in primary health care.

Months of crisis

Even before a health ministry was formed, the Sandinistas had to deal with a national crisis in health. After months of intense fighting and the virtual collapse of health services, hundreds of thousands of people urgently needed medical care.[25] Many had scarcely eaten for weeks.

Reopening hospitals and health centres was a priority. As medical supplies began to arrive at the Managua airport, some health workers also began returning to their posts. Community groups helped the effort by dismantling barricades blocking the roads and reconnecting water supplies. They also removed rubble, cleaned out bombed hospitals and health centres, and organised outpatient care.[26]

The first foreign health team to fly into Managua was a brigade of 60 Cuban doctors and nurses who arrived six days after the Sandinistas came

Chronology: 1979

17 July: Somoza flees Nicaragua for Miami.
18 July: A provisional 'Government of National Reconstruction' is established in the city of Leon. In their proclamation, they announce plans to form a 'unified national health service'.[21]
19 July: The Government of National Reconstruction takes control of Managua.
26 July: The first Cuban medical brigade arrives.[22]
1 August: The newly appointed Minister of Health asks, via *La Prensa* newspaper, that hospital directors send information on employees and their salaries. Health workers have not been paid for three to six months.
1 August: The Health Ministry announces that vaccination campaigns will be started in a few days with the help of equipment donated by the West German Government.
2 August: The Interamerican Development Bank and the Organisation of American States pledge, respectively, $20 million and $500,000 in emergency food relief.
5 August: Headline in the new *Barricada* newspaper: "The Job in Health Will Be Gigantic!"[23]
6 August: The Health Ministry announces that medical brigades have arrived from Mexico, Cuba, Germany, Panama, Costa Rica, Argentina and Honduras.[24]
10 August: The new Ministry of Health (MINSA) is inaugurated.
17 August: MINSA announcement in *La Prensa*: "The permits given to exhume cadavers of those fallen in the insurrection are suspended immediately as a hygiene measure."
20 August: The Government of Reconstruction proclaims that all INSS (social security) hospitals and clinics will be opened to the public. Private rooms in public hospitals are similarly abolished.
27 August: The Vice-Minister of Health announces: "Damage to the health system has been great, but we still don't know how great." USAID announces a further increase in aid as 2,000 tons of food arrive.
31 August: Health is proclaimed to be a right of the entire population. It is announced that there will no longer be a fee to dispense prescriptions.

to power. Within 24 hours they set up an open-air clinic next to a bombed hospital in Matagalpa. The contrast between their operation and that of the health team which played volleyball and treated Somoza supporters behind the walls of the US embassy after the 1972 earthquake could hardly have been more striking. Hundreds of patients queued up for treatment day and night. Within a month the Cuban team used up medicines which they had thought would last for three.

By late 1980 some 200 Cuban doctors and nurses were working in Nicaragua.[27] They found the experience shocking. Patients suffered from diseases such as polio and neonatal tetanus which had disappeared from Cuba. Malnutrition made the symptoms of measles so bad that the Cubans had difficulty recognising this as the same disease which, in their country, had been controlled through mass immunisation and improved nutrition. Pedro Azcuy, a member of the first Cuban health team, remembers: "I recall a very small town where there were ten or twelve children, of whom six died of measles...It was amazing to see how within ten days they began a vaccination campaign."[28]

Within months the food crisis in the cities abated. Health workers began to take services to rural areas.[29] Most nurses and doctors in Managua had never before seen or dealt with people living in rural areas. They were shocked to find people who had lived for years from hand to mouth without a roof over their heads. Concepcion Huete, later Director of Nursing, recalls:

"We went to a plantation and said: 'We are nurses from the Ministry of Health and we are here to vaccinate your children.' The people said to us: 'What is a nurse? What is vaccination?' I didn't know how to explain it to them. If somebody has never heard of a nurse, what can you tell them?"

Chapter 3:
A Health Service for All: 1979 - 1983

"The Sandinista People's Revolution...will provide free medical assistance to the entire population. It will set up clinics and hospitals throughout the national territory."
(From: *The Historic Programme of the FSLN*, 1969).[1]

Once in power, the Sandinistas moved fast. Within three weeks they inaugurated the Unified National Health System.[2] This gave the new Ministry of Health (MINSA) control over most hospitals, clinics, and the National Social Security System. It was a giant step in organisation.

The nation's new leaders were clear about the need for a national health system. They had yet to decide, however, how to make it function. What would be the roles of doctors, nurses and other health professionals? Would there be a role for private medicine? How would the public service be financed? How might community participation take shape?

These vital questions were not discussed much during the hectic weeks of 20-hour meetings in July and August 1979, when the new Government was formed. Health was awarded a high priority, but it was considered mainly a 'technical' issue, to be determined by leading revolutionary doctors.

Dr. Antonio Jarquin, one of the architects of health policy, later admitted: "The Sandinistas were specialists in destroying dictatorships, but none of us knew how to construct a government."[3] The challenge was to select strategies and technologies which would be appropriate to Nicaragua's stage of social, economic and political development. One possible model was Costa Rica, where close coordination between the social security system and the Ministry of Health, with substantial funding over a 30-year period, had brought dramatic improvements in health.[4] Also at hand was the example of Cuba, where a nationalised health service with a high concentration of doctors had raised overall health standards to the level of most industrialised countries.[5] The presence of hard-working Cuban health workers in Nicaragua also lent prestige to their model.

A massive national literacy campaign had already begun. According to Jarquin, "When you teach people to read and write you are also giving them knowledge that doctors exist, hospitals exist...it was like a bomb exploding." Nicaragua, however, had neither the time nor the funds to emulate the models of Costa Rica or Cuba.[6] Examples of simpler, less expensive health systems were put forward by the World Health Organisation, the Pan American Health Organisation, and the United Nations Children's Fund.[7] One such example was China, with its focus on health campaigns and paramedical workers known as 'barefoot doctors'. International organisations were also beginning to promote the 'primary health care' strategy (see Box).

The primary health care strategy seemed to fit well with the Sandinistas' political values and health objectives. Yet to plan and implement it throughout the country would mean overcoming enormous obstacles.

Within the Ministry of Health (MINSA), Sandinista leaders with strong trade union links argued that the health system should be oriented to the organised work force, private medicine should be completely eliminated and all health professionals should be employed by the state.

Revolutionaries who had fought in the mountains, on the other hand,

Elaborated in 1978 at a conference organised by the World Health Organisation and UNICEF at Alma Ata in the Soviet Union, primary health care was designed to make basic preventive and curative care universally available. Such care would be provided at the first level of contact with the health system. Underpinning the primary health care approach was a commitment to equity. In developing countries, this meant providing basic services for the whole population, rather than focusing on highly specialised and technologically sophisticated medical care. The specific elements of primary health care were to include:[8]

- education to prevent or control common health problems
- promotion of food supply and adequate nutrition
- safe water and basic sanitation
- maternal and child health care, including contraception
- immunisation against major diseases
- treatment of common diseases and injuries
- provision of essential drugs.

A commitment to establish universal access to these basic services was embodied in the slogan 'Health for All by the Year 2000'.

believed that the peasantry was the heart of the revolution. They argued that the new Government should give top priority to people in rural areas. Some wanted to follow China's example and down-play the role of urban hospitals and fully trained doctors. Organised medicine, for its part, favoured a 'pluralistic' approach to preserve private practice and respond to the interests of the urban middle class. New public health programmes staffed by auxiliary nurses and volunteers could be developed for the poor and rural populations.

All three groups were represented in the political coalition which brought the Sandinistas to power, and all three perspectives were represented when political compromises were made to establish a national health policy at the end of 1979.

MINSA's main focus was to be urban and rural labourers, small-scale farmers and women and children.[9] These were the groups which had fared worst under the Somoza regime. While preserving the private medical sector, MINSA would attempt to orient the entire system, including the doctors and hospitals, towards rural areas and urban slums.[10] The emphasis would be on preventive health care, health education, and community participation.[11]

This policy contained the seeds of conflict. On one hand, the Government proclaimed the need for low-cost, community-based, preventive health services. On the other hand, it also promised to provide wide access to curative care in modern hospitals. This well-intentioned commitment was inconsistent with the primary health care approach. It was medically inappropriate and financially overwhelming. Yet pressure from the population and a belief that the 'best' care should be available to all made this political choice inevitable.

These contradictory views led to lively and sometimes acrimonious debates in MINSA. A leading opponent of the high-tech, hospital-based approach was Dr. Adolfo Chamorro. A military commander during the revolutionary war, Dr. Chamorro helped initiate a paramedical programme involving 15,000 volunteers in the country's national literacy campaign of 1980.[12] He also advocated workers' health schemes as part of self-management.[13] Frustrated with both the government bureaucracy and the conservatism of the medical establishment, Dr. Chamorro went back to the army when the *Contra* war intensified in 1982. As one of Chamorro's supporters later reflected: "Adolfo was just ahead of his time."

Reaching the people

After 1979 doctors and nurses suddenly arrived in rural and poor urban communities. But this expression of the Government's commitment to equity in health also brought complications. Dr. Leonel Arguello did his social service in the remote Atlantic Coast town of Rama in 1980:

"Peasants would walk for days to reach the town because they had heard that there was a doctor. But they had no idea what to do when they got there. They would stand silently, with stoic pride, on the other side of the path in front of the clinic. If I didn't go out to ask them about their problems and invite them into the clinic, they would simply return home after a few days. They still weren't convinced that they had a right to health care."

Another young doctor, Roberto Valle Gonzalez, summed up the situation with a touch of wry humour: "We feel a need to rescue them from their backwardness, but they don't necessarily see this the same way we do."

Soon, however, even in remote areas, confidence in the new health services grew and they were used *en masse*. In the towns and cities, the demand for free health care created early morning queues at clinics that

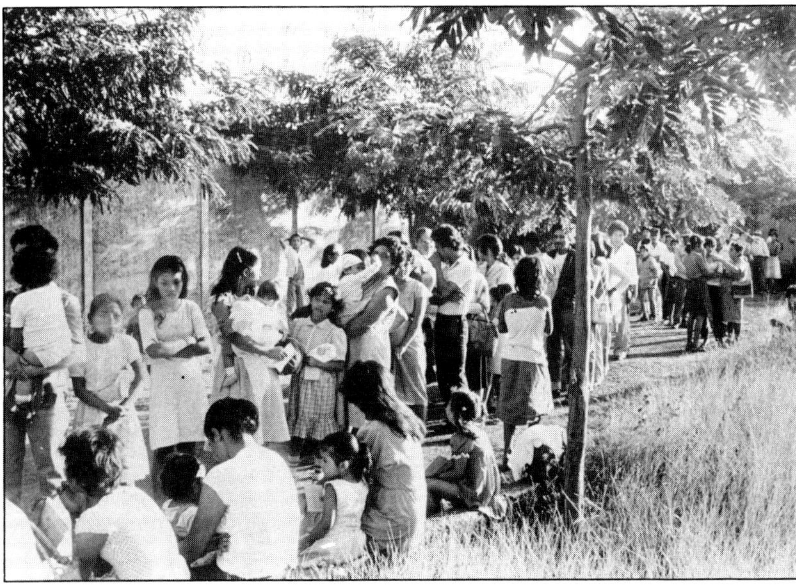

E BARRETO / BARRICADA

The new health services proved very popular. Scene at 6 a.m. outside a health centre, in 1983.

snaked down the street in the hot sun as far as the eye could see. Hospitals were also deluged with patients. Alta Hooker worked as a nurse in the regional hospital of the Atlantic Coast town of Puerto Cabezas:

"Before the revolution, we never filled the 27 beds in the hospital. About two months after the war of liberation, I attended a two-month anaesthesia course in Managua. When I got back I found lots of sickness in and around the hospital, because the people were really starting to come in. It became impossible to work — you'd nearly walk on the patients lying on stretchers or on the ground between beds. The Ministry of Health told us that we'd have to be patient, that it was the same everywhere, and we'd just have to wait our turn. We increased the number of beds from 27 to 69 in that first year, and in 1985 we got a new wing with 22 more beds."

This new access to care brought out a shocking legacy of long neglect. Dr. Antonio Dager examined a woman who had what appeared to be a growth the size of a volleyball on her abdomen.[14] She said that it had been the size of a marble 15 years before, and now caused her to vomit constantly. "What could it be? If it was intestine, she shouldn't be vomiting. If it was strangulated she would have died years ago. The books didn't help at all." It turned out that her entire stomach was in a hernia outside her abdominal muscles. Her recovery was uneventful after a simple operation.

Frenetic building

The years 1979-1981 were marked by frenetic construction of new health facilities. In 1979 there were fewer than 200 health centres and health posts in the country. This was far too few for the Sandinistas to fulfil their promise of providing services in isolated areas. A massive building programme was needed, but some advised caution. Dr. Giorgio Solimano, a Chilean who had worked in the Health Ministry of the Allende Government in Chile, was one of these:

"The people's expectations were enormous and grew day by day, fuelled by pronouncements by officials of the new Government. How they were going to meet those expectations was anybody's guess."

By 1982 more than 300 new health posts had been built.[15] This provided the physical infrastructure needed for primary health care throughout the country[16] (see Figure 3.1). Only about half of these new facilities were constructed by the Government. The remainder were built by communities themselves. Dr. Leonel Arguello helped to build the health post in the Atlantic Coast township of Punta Gorda:

"Before the revolution, the Moravian church was used for all types of social functions, and once a year a pastor came to perform weddings and baptisms. We started by giving medical attention in the church as well, and then talked to the people about how it would be to have a clinic. One person brought his boat to transport materials. Another offered his services as a carpenter. Doctors, nurses, and the community people did the labour. Whenever we ran short of materials, people put out a call for donations or raised money to buy what was needed."

In many places existing buildings were converted into health centres or posts. In the town of El Cua a notorious prison was converted into a health centre with beds. In many small towns the elegant homes of Somoza supporters who had fled the country in 1979 were turned into spacious health centres. One of Managua's better-designed health centres

Fig. 3.1

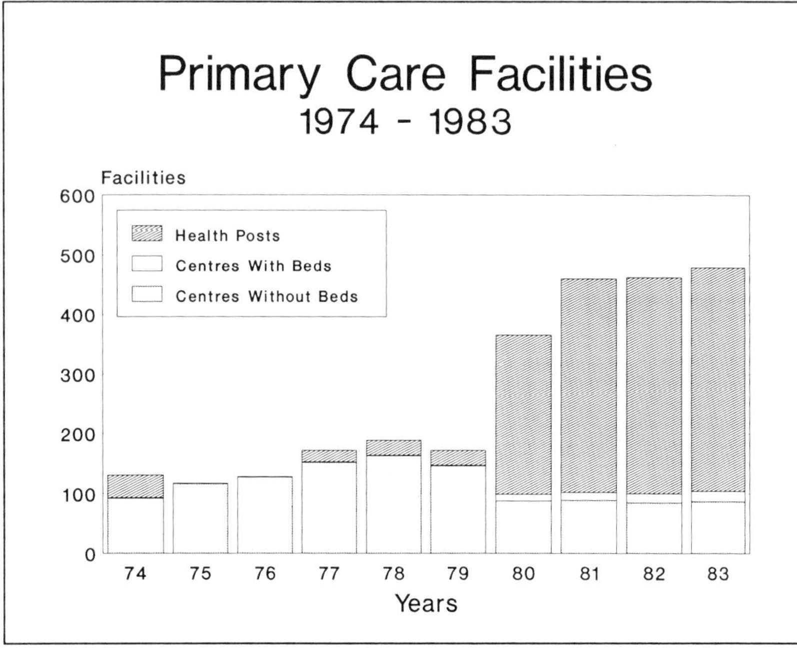

The number of health facilities rose rapidly immediately after the revolution as new health posts were established.

was once a brothel owned by one of Somoza's colonels.[17] When the revolutionary Government proposed turning it into a prison, community groups persuaded the Government that the building, with its rows of small cubicles, would be put to better use for medical consultations.[18]

Where health centres or posts could not be set up, mobile units, moving by truck or boat, visited weekly.[19] MINSA was not alone in this effort. Newly established state farms were assigned health workers who served as focal points for care to peasants living in the area.[20] Social security clinics and hospitals, formerly restricted to insured workers, were also opened to the general public. With the huge surge in building, the Government's biggest task became staffing these facilities.

Training for rural health

In many remote parts of the country, the first health workers to arrive were young volunteers *(brigadistas)* with only two weeks' training in health care. Beginning just eight months after the Sandinistas came to power, the National Literacy Campaign recruited close to 100,000 volunteers — mostly high school and university students — to teach basic literacy skills to 400,000 adults between March and September of 1980.[21] MINSA trained 15,000 of these literacy *brigadistas* in first aid, sanitation, and malaria and diarrhoea control at the newly formed Polytechnic Institute in Managua.[22] Apart from teaching literacy skills, these young men and women also worked as rural health aides, collected information on local herbal medicines and folk healing practices, and helped to construct health posts.

When the literacy campaign ended, the Polytechnic Institute began to train thousands of auxiliary nurses as well as laboratory and dental technicians. The Institute was unprepared for this task, and students received instruction in open pavilions while the walls were being built.[23]

Meanwhile, medical students near the end of their courses were rushed into service, doubling the number of new graduates in 1980 and 1981. A second medical school in Managua was opened to help reach the target of 500 new doctors a year by 1985.

Professional nurses were trained in similarly shortened courses, so that by 1981 their numbers had also increased. But the greatest increase in health personnel occurred among auxiliary nurses, who were trained *en masse* between 1979 and 1982 in nine or twelve-month courses. During this period the numbers being trained increased five-fold.[24]

A rational health system

Building a rational health system on the imbalanced base of existing facilities was a daunting task. It was made doubly difficult when health officials of the old regime were encouraged to stay on. In a reconciliatory gesture and to avoid the loss of personnel with rare administrative skills, only the highest or most corrupt health officials were dismissed.

It took MINSA several months just to determine how many clinics and hospital beds existed. Health officials worked with three different estimates of the number of doctors in the country. As the organisational dust settled, a three-tiered national health structure emerged (see Box).

The Structure of Health Care

The health service in 1980 was reorganised according to the three levels of technical sophistication of its institutions: hospitals, health centres, and health posts.[25] This system is still largely in place.

The most technologically advanced care is provided at seven national-level hospitals in Managua and Leon and three foreign-run hospitals in Managua and Chinandega. These include surgical, paediatric, and gynaecological specialty hospitals. Other nationally-run hospitals include those providing long-term residential care for patients with leprosy or other skin diseases, tuberculosis, rehabilitation needs, or psychiatric problems.

The system is subdivided into six regions and the Zelaya Autonomous Zone on the Atlantic coast. The regions administer 20 'secondary care'

Structure of the Public Health System

Administration	Population	Facilities	Personnel and Services
Nation	3,600,000	National Referral Hospitals (14)	Rehabilitation Specialty and Subspecialty Care
Region (6)	10,000 – 100,000	Regional Hospitals (16)	Surgery and Basic Specialties
Area (97)	5000 – 20,000	Health Centre or Post (104)	Graduate Nurse and Basic Specialties: Gynaecology Paediatrics Internal Medicine Obstetrics
Sector (500)	1000 – 3000	Post or Community Centre (417)	Visiting Doctors Auxiliary Nurse Malaria Worker Brigadistas Health Educator

hospitals staffed mainly by social service physicians and foreign volunteers. They usually have local community doctors and specialists as well. A doctor is present 24 hours a day. Eight of Nicaragua's nine private hospitals and the 23 private clinics with beds are also at this level of technical sophistication. Nine of the best regional hospitals are also teaching units with newly-qualified doctors and medical students working in them.

Within the regions and autonomous zone are health areas. Each region contains 10-20 health areas. The country has a total of 97 health areas, each covering 20,000-30,000 people. Primary care is provided at health centres and health posts in the areas.

Health centres are found in larger villages, towns, and cities of 5,000-15,000 residents. Patients can be referred to a health centre from a health post, but most come on their own. There is at least one doctor present whenever the centre is open. Health centres provide gynaecological, paediatric and internal medicine, and obstetric care. Larger centres may have four or more doctors, including older local physicians who work part-time and specialists who visit periodically. Some laboratory services are available, some clinics have a pharmacy, and a few even have X-ray

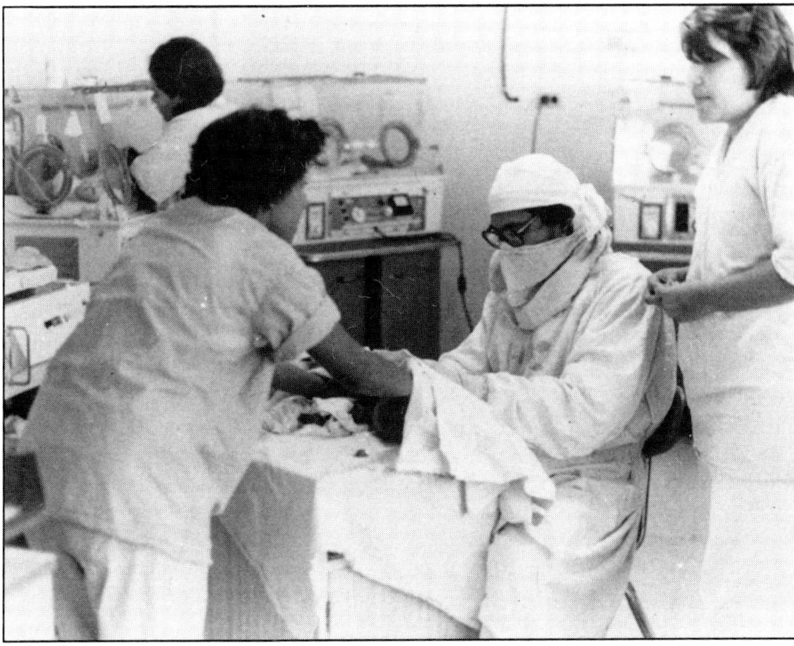

The intensive care unit for newborn babies at Berta Calderon Hospital in Managua. Sophisticated health-care technology is available in a few Nicaraguan hospitals.

machines. Many offer dental services and some have beds for overnight care.

Health posts are usually located in villages with less than 5,000 residents, though there are several posts in the city of Managua. Rural posts are usually staffed by a nurse or auxiliary nurse and are visited once or twice a week by a doctor. They deal with common illnesses, prenatal check-ups, well-child visits, and minor first aid. A post usually doubles as an oral rehydration centre. There is no clinical laboratory, although in some posts laboratory samples can be taken. In the most remote parts of the country health volunteers provide basic care in makeshift clinics or out of a knapsack.

A health post or centre functions as the nucleus for health activities in the *area*. Each *area* employs a health educator. The key to local health promotion is the subdivision of the *area* served by the health centre or post into three to six *sectors*. Each *sector* has 1,000-2,000 residents, is served by an auxiliary nurse and one or more local health aides, and is supervised by a physician at the health centre. The auxiliary nurse monitors community health, helps coordinate and promote health campaigns, and provides preventive care to people in the sector.

Problem hospitals

When the Sandinistas came to power, work had begun on four of five new hospitals designed and financed by USAID. Work ground to a halt, however, when USAID funding tapered off in 1980 and stopped altogether in 1981. Signs with the familiar handshake logo and the inscription 'Funded by the people of the United States' were removed from the construction sites and the Nicaraguan Government took responsibility for further construction.

These new hospitals were seen as symbols of the Government's commitment to provide health care for all. Their completion was therefore a matter of great political importance. Unfortunately, serious errors in planning and construction resulted in long delays. The new hospital in Bluefields, on the Atlantic Coast, was built by a foreign construction firm which failed to include the contracted structural supports under the building. By the time the hospital was due to open in 1985, it was already sinking into the sandy soil. Its opening was delayed for a year and construction costs doubled while necessary improvements were made.

The Matagalpa Hospital, designed as a large modern complex with a commanding view of the city, was situated so far from residential areas that new bus routes had to be established to make it accessible. When it was found that the municipal water system lacked pressure to raise water to the hilltop site, the opening was postponed for 12 months to allow for the construction of a new water system.

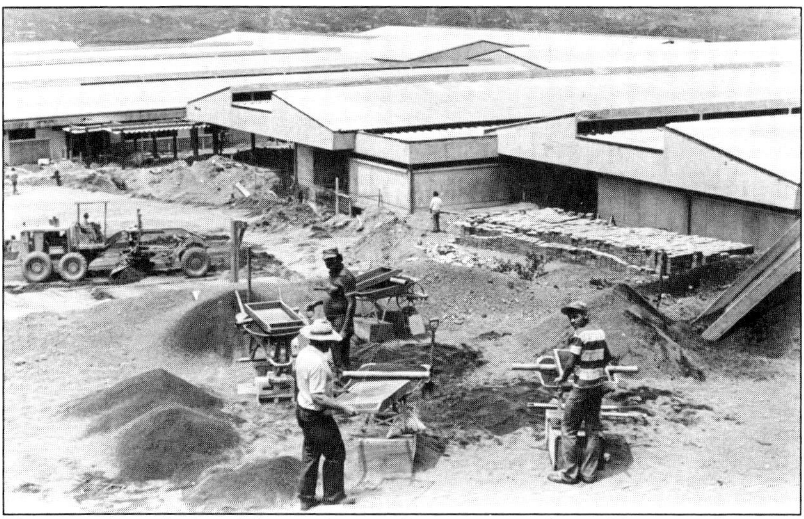

BARRICADA

The new hospital at Matagalpa under construction. The opening was delayed because of the need for a new water system. This hospital was one of those originally designed by USAID.

Fig. 3.2

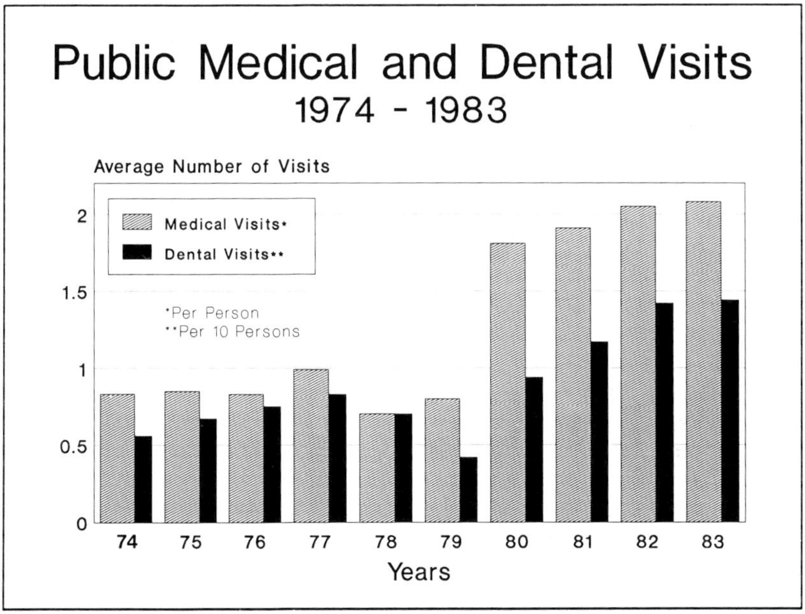

Per capita medical and dental visits fell during the years of the insurrection and rose rapidly following the revolution. These data are for public institutions; no data are available on private medical and dental consultations.

Reducing inequalities

As large numbers of health workers were trained and assigned to facilities in rural areas, geographic inequalities decreased dramatically. In 1980, Managua had one doctor for every 1,000 people, while in some remote regions there was a doctor for every 10,000 residents. The gap in geographic coverage of nurses was also huge. The best-endowed region had one graduate nurse per 3,000 residents; the worst region had one nurse per 20,000 people. These enormous variations in distribution were reduced rapidly after 1979.[26] By 1983 the best and worst health regions had only a two-fold difference in coverage of nurses and doctors.

The growth in access was most dramatic for basic curative medical care. In 1971, 12% of the country's doctors, 11% of the nurses, and 9% of the auxiliary nurses worked in primary care. By 1981, as a result of the large influx of health workers into rural areas after July 1979, 36% of the doctors, 30% of the nurses, and 30% of the auxiliaries — including almost all new graduates — worked in primary care.

Public health programmes for rural areas, maternal and child health, and occupational medicine expanded enormously after 1979. Outpatient care and prescriptions — the curative services most lacking for the general population prior to 1979 — showed the most dramatic increases. From 1977 to 1983, hospitalisations and surgical procedures rose more than 50%, outpatient medical visits tripled (see Figure 3.2), and the number of vaccinations increased more than four-fold.

By 1982, at least 70% of the population received some medical care from trained staff. This was a dramatic increase over the 28% receiving modern health care prior to 1979.[27] The average number of visits to a doctor more than doubled. Northern Zelaya zone on the Atlantic Coast had the highest rate of doctor visits, with more than three consultations per capita each year. Nonetheless, towns and cities were still better served than most rural areas. Residents of Managua in 1982 averaged 55% more medical consultations than people in the rest of the country.

Losers under the new system

This meteoric expansion in services may hide the fact that for some groups the revolution meant poorer access to health care. The most obvious of these groups was the rich. They no longer enjoyed private beds at the major government hospitals. This was not greatly missed. When not seriously ill, the rich still had private clinics and hospitals to cater for their needs. When seriously ill, they generally went to Miami or Houston for care. The advent of the revolution simply made this option relatively more attractive.

The middle class also lost privileged access to care following 1979. The poor might be content to wait hours in the sun to see a doctor at a government health centre. The middle class was not, and began visiting private doctors. Yet even private medicine was subject to shortages of equipment and supplies. Amid complaints about empty pharmacy shelves, relatives and friends living abroad were increasingly relied on for medicines unobtainable in Nicaragua.

The largest and most powerful group to lose preferential access was the unionised work force. Representing about 26,000 people before 1979, union ranks swelled to more than 100,000 in 1980. The single largest organised group of workers was composed of government employees, who represented about a third of the unionised work force. Many unions opposed the opening of social security clinics and hospitals to the general public, because this would entail a rapid decline in the amount and quality of care which they could obtain for their members. Unions repeatedly petitioned the Government to re-establish preferential access to care.

Although unions were given minor concessions for several months, their privileged system of care was not re-established and workers threatened to strike. In the end, however, opposition faded because so many trade unionists depended directly or indirectly on the Government for their income.

For several years the Ministry of Agriculture continued to operate an independent health service on state-owned farms. It was only in 1983 that the last social security hospital, at the Ingenio Julio Butriago sugar mill, was finally brought under direct MINSA control.

Health leaders

The first Minister of Health was a respected paediatric neurosurgeon, Dr. Cesar Amador Kuhl. The selection of Dr. Kuhl, a political independent popular with most doctors, seemed a cautious step for a revolutionary government. His political neutrality, however, made him more acceptable to people from a wide political spectrum, both within and outside the country. He brought unity to the new Ministry and played a leading role in obtaining international assistance. But his lack of political and administrative expertise put him in a weak position to lead such a complex government ministry. In early 1981 Dr. Kuhl returned to private practice, university teaching, and leadership of the *Colegio de Medicos*.[28]

His successor was Lea Guido, a 32-year-old Sandinista activist and Lecturer in Sociology who had studied at the University of Lausanne in Switzerland. Ms. Guido had led the national women's organisation, and was the new Government's first Minister of Social Welfare in 1979. She had no medical qualifications but was known as an effective administrator.

Although her youth was no bar to such a high office, she had to operate in an environment in which *machismo* still flourished and conservative medical attitudes were deeply ingrained. Inevitably, her appointment caused consternation among doctors, who feared political interference in medicine. The stage was set for a trial of strength between a Sandinista Health Minister and the medical establishment. Much of this battle would be fought over issues concerning community involvement in health.

Chapter 4: Community Participation

"I don't know much about science, but a doctor doesn't know this neighbourhood like I do. When we work together, the doctor and I can make democracy a reality in health. But democracy isn't always easy."
(Rosa Garcia, health volunteer)

A solid basis for community participation in health was laid during the revolutionary insurrections of 1978 and 1979, when Civil Defence Committees had taken over responsibility for health administration in some areas. But when the Sandinistas came to power in July 1979, they had yet to formulate a plan for community participation in health. How could participation be organised so that it was genuinely local and spontaneous, rather than imposed from above? How could such participation be spread throughout the whole health system? And would the people want to participate anyway? These were questions to which there were no ready-made answers.[1]

There was to be no return to the token participation of the 1970s. A national programme to involve traditional birth attendants (TBAs) in family planning and health care, for example, had failed because of a lack of community interest and involvement. Corruption and poor leadership had resulted in high costs and poor efficiency in a USAID-sponsored sanitation project, where administrative costs amounted to 60% of the total budget.[2] Some of these programmes were little more than window dressing for an unpopular regime. Several were located in areas of high guerrilla activity in order to collect strategic military information. All suffered from a lack of credibility and community involvement because of the narrow interests they represented and the unpopular political regime they served.[3]

Attempts to mobilise the population after July 1979 began with the most pressing concerns of the people. The first organised activities involved food distribution and the most successful vaccination campaign in the nation's history, achieving 70% coverage against polio in some areas. Measles and diphtheria-pertussis-tetanus vaccination programmes soon followed.

The immunisation campaign also brought to light the limited understanding people had of diseases and their prevention. Many parents were suspicious and refused to bring their children to vaccination posts. Some, never having seen a doctor or nurse, and fearing that injections would make their children ill, simply hid from vaccination teams.

It became clear that massive public education was needed.[4] Families needed to learn about immunisation, sanitation, nutrition and common diseases. But how could large numbers of barely literate people be motivated to learn about health? In 1980, MINSA experimented with teams of health educators who promoted 'health literacy' by using socio-drama, role-play, puppetry and participatory theatre. The task turned out to be far beyond the capacity of these small teams. A method was urgently needed for training large numbers of community members in a short period of time. Once trained, these people could then spread health knowledge and organise their communities to carry out activities to prevent diseases.

The National Literacy Crusade of 1980 provided a possible model. The Crusade had trained a core group of literacy teachers, who in turn trained tens of thousands more through a 'multiplier' strategy in which each trained volunteer in turn became a trainer of others. Adapting this strategy to its own needs, MINSA trained 100 health educators, then 1,000 'multipliers', and finally 30,000 health volunteers, called *brigadistas*.[5] The *brigadistas* made house-to-house visits and gave small-group talks to educate and motivate their neighbours in health matters. In a little over a year, thousands of health volunteers were active in neighbourhoods and villages throughout the country[6] (see Figure 4.1).

To support this massive effort, the Ministry of Health (MINSA) developed illustrated, comic-style booklets. According to a training manual, the objective was to develop "content and methods which corresponded to popular needs, [making education] a liberating process".[7] Booklets were printed on newsprint paper and distributed throughout the country. They covered a wide range of topics including immunisation, hygiene and sanitation, rabies, tuberculosis, breastfeeding, first-aid, nutrition, diarrhoea, dental care, food handling, water supply and insect control.

Designed to promote an understanding of the causes, prevention and treatment of major illnesses, the booklets also related health problems to their social and political context.[8] The booklet on breastfeeding, for example, discussed the role of international corporations in promoting powdered milk, as well as the cultural biases which downgrade breastfeeding as 'uneducated'. The booklets were widely used by neighbourhood and church groups, trade unions, cooperatives, women's groups, literacy classes and schools.

Fig. 4.1

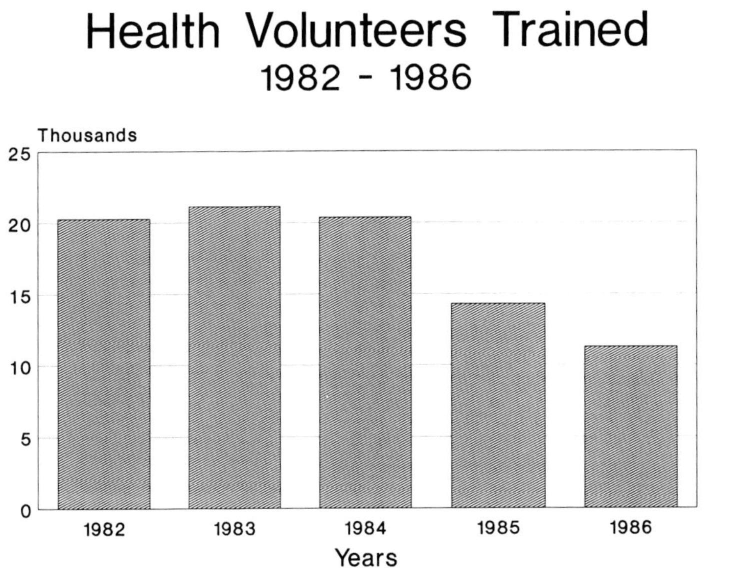

The number of volunteers being trained to take part in health campaigns declined by 1985 as many experienced volunteers avoided repeated training. No data are available on the total numbers of volunteers active in the country after 1982.

Health educators and *brigadistas* studied the booklets in groups in order to stimulate discussion and analysis of health problems. By 1988 over two dozen different booklets had been produced and more than 3 million copies had been distributed.

As more experience was gained with health campaigns, and as local groups gained the self-confidence to criticise national programmes, it became clear that the original booklets had serious limitations.[9] The drawings, for example, were too abstract for many *campesinos*, and the handwritten texts often proved illegible to people who had only recently learned to read. Simpler drawings and typewritten texts were used in subsequent booklets.

The release of a booklet was often timed to coincide with the popularisation of a health slogan and with a practical action. Radio, television, newspapers and other media were used to promote health messages. The prevention and treatment of diarrhoea — the single most common cause of child death — was a focus of particular attention. Special programmes and advertising 'spots' on radio and television

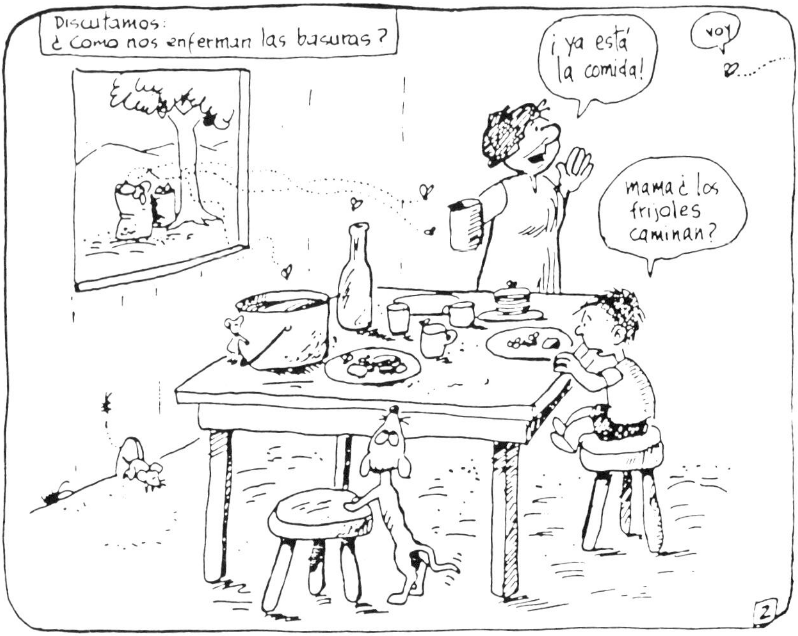
Discutamos:
¿Como nos enferman las basuras?
¡ya está la comida!
voy
mama ¿los frijoles caminan?
2

Pamphlets of this kind were found to be too complicated and hard to read. A simpler pamphlet (below) with typewritten words was more effective.

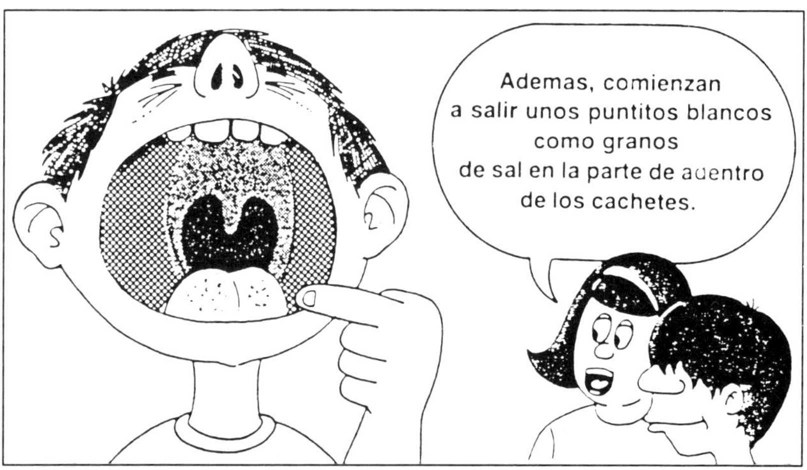
Ademas, comienzan a salir unos puntitos blancos como granos de sal en la parte de adentro de los cachetes.

explained the causes and dangers of diarrhoea, and what families themselves could do to prevent and treat the disease.

Roadside billboards, newspaper comic strips and advertisements, and posters in health centres were also widely used. The first slogan concerning diarrhoea was: "A child with diarrhoea can die. Take yours to the nearest oral rehydration* centre (URO)". UROs were started by community groups in community centres or private homes in 1979. Within 12 months over 200 such units had been set up. Most were run by a health volunteer or a nursing auxiliary (see also Chapter 9).

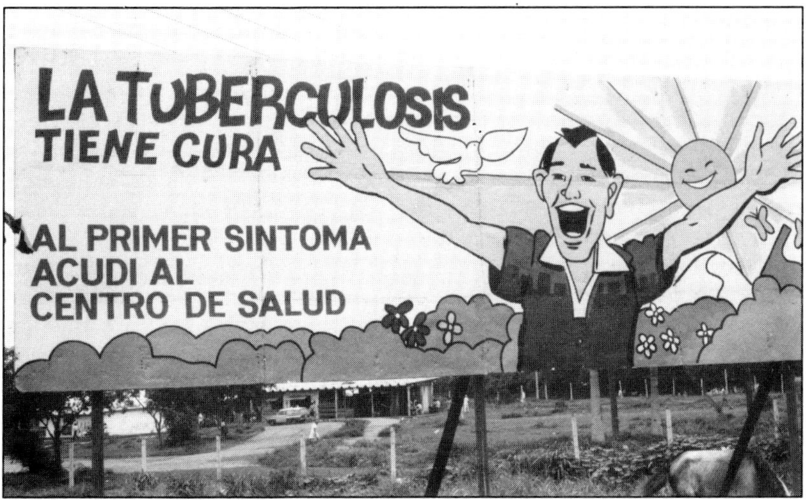
LA TUBERCULOSIS
TIENE CURA
AL PRIMER SINTOMA
ACUDI AL
CENTRO DE SALUD

NICARAGUA HEALTH FUND

Roadside billboard: "Tuberculosis has a cure. Go to the health centre at the first symptom".

People's Health Councils

Education for health action required a system for involving communities in planning, implementation and evaluation. In July 1980 the Government established People's Health Councils in order to "mould the aspirations of the people into concrete programmes" and "channel the activities and concerns of the people in a coordinated manner".[10]

The first health councils consisted only of representatives of community organisations.[11] The most important of these were neighbourhood associations known as Sandinista Defence Committees (CDS). Also active were the national women's organisation (AMNLAE), the farm labourers' union (ATC), the workers' union (CST), the teachers' union (UNE), the youth movement (JS19S), the children's association (ASN) and the health workers' union (FETSALUD).

Some of these organisations — especially the Sandinista Defence Committees — were already involved in organising health campaigns and carrying out health education.[12] Previously, however, their involvement had been unofficial, spontaneous, and seemingly anarchic in character.

*** Oral Rehydration Therapy is the administration of fluid by mouth to prevent or treat the dehydration caused by diarrhoea.**

Through community health councils these organisations were recognised as having the right — and the responsibility — to participate in health matters.

Councils were established at local, regional and national levels to parallel official MINSA structures. The councils took responsibility for organising campaigns known as 'People's Health Days' to combat particular health problems.[13] In 1980, for example, an estimated 30,000 volunteers took part in a series of Health Days focusing on polio, measles, dengue and environmental sanitation. On each occasion, volunteers attended weekend training sessions and made door-to-door visits to explain the purpose of the forthcoming Health Day. For the immunisation campaigns, the volunteers also carried out a census of infants and children in their neighbourhood who required vaccination. Each campaign was followed by 'Analysis and Summary' meetings involving doctors, nurses and health volunteers.

In 1981, the councils mounted four major campaigns: a campaign against polio and measles, an environmental sanitation campaign, an anti-dengue campaign, and — most ambitious of all — an anti-malaria campaign involving about 200,000 voluntary workers[14] (see Chapter 5). Within MINSA, the department dealing with campaigns, the Division for Education and Popular Communication for Health (DECOPS), became so large and active that other, more conservative sections of MINSA were alarmed. It was even feared that DECOPS might take over the Division of Preventive Medicine.

Both conservatives and radicals were concerned about the meteoric growth in health campaign activities. Conservatives lacked trust in the *brigadista* programme because it threatened to replace professional medicine as the heart of the health system. Radicals were concerned that volunteer activity might take pressure off the efforts to reorient medicine toward the poor majority. The 'appropriate technology' of volunteers and preventive campaigns might thus leave doctors free to continue 'business as usual' with their urban, middle-class clientele.

Organised communities

Sandinista Defence Committees (CDSs) are usually the most active community groups. A CDS at the level of the urban 'block' or rural neighbourhood consists of 50-200 people. A group of about ten blocks makes up a *barrio*, and about five *barrios* make up a zone of the national CDS organisation.[15] Most blocks and neighbourhoods have a CDS: as many as 8,000 CDSs have functioned at the zonal level, covering about 75% of all urban neighbourhoods in the country.

Rural CDSs often have two subcommittees: one for welfare (including health) and another for production and defence. More elaborate urban CDSs have had as many as five subcommittees: organisation, defence, education, health, and production. A local CDS may organise health activities as it sees fit. Locally initiated campaigns include environmental clean-ups, first-aid training, civil defence drills, and — in isolated areas — the training of volunteer paramedical health workers. A CDS may be involved in many health-related activities (see Box).

Health activities of a Sandinista Defence Committee

Celine Woznica, a Maryknoll missioner, was working in Ciudad Sandino during the mid-1980s. She reported on some activities of the Sandinista Defence Committee (CDS) at that time:

- **Social support:**[16] Don Lencho, an elderly man suffering from leg ulcers and unable to care for himself, lived alone. A CDS meeting decided to ask a physician to examine him. The doctor explained that Don Lencho's poor health was due more to isolation than medical causes. In response CDS families took turns preparing an extra plate of food for the old man at mealtimes. A nurse from the clinic also came to his house to dress his ulcers — a job later taken over by a local health volunteer.
- **Disaster relief:**[17] When a flash flood washed away 60 homes and damaged 160 others, the CDS evacuated families to local churches and school buildings, distributed food and clothing, and successfully petitioned the Government for new plots of land and permission to build new houses.
- **Community health services:**[18] When the Evangelical Church set up an Oral Rehydration Unit, the CDS recruited six health volunteers from each of the zones to help staff it.
- **Distribution of consumer goods:**[19] Among the many consumer goods in short supply were baby bottles and nappies, resulting in exorbitant prices for these items on the black market. The CDS persuaded the Ministry of Interior Commerce to make them available at guaranteed prices for women who brought their prenatal cards to the government distribution stores. This action resulted in 60% higher attendance of pregnant women at the prenatal clinic.
- **Sanitation:**[20] A single mother with several young children, living in a shack with no latrine, was reduced to using a chamber pot to empty family waste in a neighbour's latrine. Upon hearing that MINSA would give the base and seat of a latrine to anyone willing to dig the hole, the CDS decided to help the woman. One Sunday morning, a group of volunteers dug a hole, installed the latrine and constructed a small shed to provide privacy for the woman and her family.

The volunteers

Despite the wide popularity of the new Government, many people wanted to avoid direct political involvement. Participation in health was a less overt, and therefore more acceptable, way to help rebuild the country. To political leaders, on the other hand, volunteer health activities were a way of attracting people into a commitment to the revolution's social and political goals.

Rosa Garcia's story is typical.[21] In September 1978 she gave refuge in her home to a young guerrilla fleeing Somoza's National Guard. Soon she opened a stand near the entrance to Ciudad Sandino where she sold fruit drinks. There she observed the movements of the National Guard, chatted with the Guardsmen who purchased drinks from her, and later passed the information on to the FSLN. She had always been interested in health, but at the age of 28 she was still illiterate. She learned to read in the National Literacy Crusade in 1980 and became active as a health *brigadista*. In the following year she led sanitation and anti-malarial campaigns in her neighbourhood. In 1982 her neighbours chose her to coordinate local health activities and represent them on the board of the health centre.

Like Rosa Garcia, most *brigadistas* are part-time activists. Their work is greatest immediately before and during the 'People's Health Days' which are usually held four times a year. They come from a wide spectrum of Nicaraguan society. A survey of the 30,000 volunteers trained for a sanitation campaign in 1982 found that most were young:[22] 75% were under 25 years of age, and 20% under 15. Although most were literate, only a minority had finished primary school. This pattern continues today. At least two-thirds of *brigadistas* are women; most of them are urban housewives or students.[23] Most male *brigadistas* are rural farmers or urban students. About 20% of all *brigadistas* are either salaried workers or self-employed.

The drop-out rate among part-time health *brigadistas* is high, due to the large amount of time and effort demanded by the 'Health Days'. Many volunteers are students, who move, marry, or take full-time jobs. After participating in campaigns for several years, many volunteers lose their enthusiasm. Especially with the decline in living standards of recent years, the demands of day-to-day survival make voluntarism more difficult.

Recruitment and training methods for part-time health *brigadistas* have gradually changed.[24] Until 1983, they were recruited and trained separately for each campaign. This method proved inefficient. Many *brigadistas* had been trained in previous campaigns and already had the necessary skills and experience. There were also frequent conflicts between the need for volunteers for the health campaigns and other mobilisation efforts such as coffee-harvesting, tree-planting, community clean-ups and participation in local militias.[25] In addition, the expanding

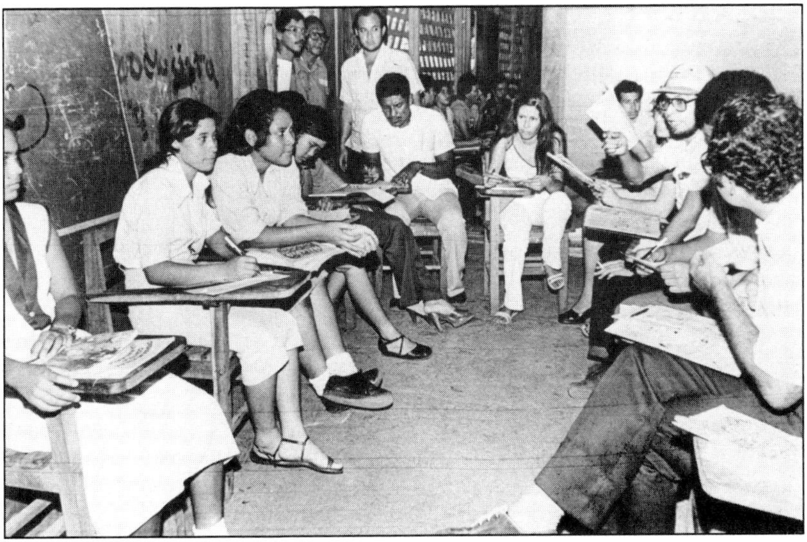

E BARRETO / BARRICADA

Training workshop for volunteers in a health campaign, 1981.

health system was reducing the need for some of the original functions of *brigadistas*.

In response, MINSA began to provide more intensive, on-going training. Fewer are now being trained (see Figure 4.1), but most are trained for one or two weeks in order to take extended responsibilities, rather than trained for only one day for short-term campaigns as before. Some are also being trained to treat common infections and other illnesses. In addition, MINSA provides *brigadistas* with non-monetary rewards such as scholarships, identification badges and diplomas to give them greater status in the community.

Some critics argue that this is still not enough. Ana Quiros, from the non-governmental health education group CISAS, believes that more responsibility and training should have been given to the *brigadistas* when the war escalated in 1983. "That was the moment to strengthen community participation, not neglect it."[26]

Remuneration for health volunteers, in cash or in kind, remains a controversial issue. Some believe it is unreasonable to ask volunteers to work for years without some type of payment. The dominant view within MINSA, however, is that paying *brigadistas* would be an untenable financial burden. It would also undermine the spirit of voluntarism which has helped to stimulate widespread community participation.

In the south of the Atlantic coast area, however, the sparse population, difficult terrain and lack of communications means that there is a clear need for full-time paramedical workers at community level. The regional

MINSA office trains full-time health *brigadistas* to provide curative and preventive health services.[27] These *brigadistas* use canoes as 'ambulances' to ferry seriously ill patients to health centres, and are relatively well-supplied with basic medicines despite shortages at many health centres and hospitals. This is in marked contrast to the situation in many other developing countries, where the community health worker is at the end of the supply chain and loses credibility because of a lack of basic drugs and supplies.

Who decides?

Community participation involves more than labour for 'Health Days'. Above all, it means having a say in what sort of health care is made available.[28] This was one of the main reasons for establishing People's Health Councils in 1980. In 1981 the membership of Health Councils was broadened to include health professionals — a decision that many feel has discouraged autonomous community initiative. Maryknoll missioner Celine Woznica lived in Ciudad Sandino at that time. Later, she summed up her concern as follows:[29]

"The over-riding problem with the People's Health Councils is the dominance of the Ministry of Health. This stands in the way of broad and effective community participation."

Lacking the authority and funds for independent initiatives, many community health leaders feel weak in relation to doctors and health officials. Guillermo Sanchez, a former school teacher, became a full-time health organiser in Esteli:

"We want our communities to be healthy, so we carry out health campaigns. But the local doctor where I live doesn't like it — he feels we are taking his business away or showing disrespect for his position. I have to take this into consideration, because he is the only doctor in the area. What will I do if my children fall ill and he won't provide treatment? And what if the doctor goes to Managua or leaves the country? Even a reactionary doctor is better than no doctor at all."

Many community leaders, however, feel less inhibited by the authority of local officials and doctors. When communities take charge of their health care, conflicts are inevitable. In Ciudad Sandino, for example, the local CDS repeatedly asked the health centre director to replace the ambulance which broke down beyond repair in 1982.[30] But the director refused to pass on the request to MINSA, giving as his reason the lack of personnel to run the ambulance or determine which patients genuinely needed its services. Two years later, to the director's great annoyance, the CDS took its request directly to the regional MINSA office.

Dissociating himself from the request, the director decided instead to seek funds and authority for the construction of a small hospital for mothers and children. This proposal, however, was rejected by MINSA as too costly. Community leaders were finally able to put their request directly to the President and the Minister of Health during a televised, open-air 'face the people' session in 1984. This bold move eventually resulted in the health centre receiving a new ambulance donated by a foreign organisation. Two years later, an obstetrics wing was added to the health centre.

Financial conflicts are common. In 1981, for example, the CDS of Ciudad Sandino decided to collect one *cordoba* as a 'voluntary contribution' from patients waiting to see a physician.[31] The purpose of these collections was to buy medical equipment, construct benches and chairs, and support community health activities. Because the policy of the Government was to provide health care without charge, the CDS obtained special permission from the Ministry of Health for these collections. By 1983, such collections had become common in many parts of the country.

In 1984, however, the regional MINSA office ordered the CDS to stop collecting money from patients.[32] With national elections scheduled for November of that year, the official policy of free health care assumed greater political importance, over-riding the issue of local autonomy. The CDS in Ciudad Sandino did not challenge the directive even though it meant the loss of its only regular source of income. Left out of the decision-making process, the CDS slipped into a more passive role. Attendance of *brigadistas* at CDS meetings fell off and more dropped out of community health activities. Similar dynamics occurred when community groups lost control over MINSA-owned weighing scales used for well-baby checkups and food supplement distribution.

The war on participation

The country's economic troubles are probably not as great a deterrent to participation as is the war. In the war zones, hundreds of *brigadistas* and community leaders have stopped volunteering for fear of reprisals by the *Contras* (see Chapter 6). In 1983, as the *Contra* rebels increased their attacks on the civilian population, community participation moved onto a war footing.

Many People's Health Councils, especially in areas directly affected by the *Contra* war, trained *brigadistas* in first-aid. When petroleum storage tanks in the port of Corinto were set ablaze by a *Contra* attack, *brigadistas* were able to treat the injured and help to organise a rapid evacuation. In areas where *Contra* activity makes it dangerous for families to travel to health facilities, *brigadistas* carry out immunisation on a house-to-house basis. They play a leading role in preventing or containing outbreaks of diseases such as diarrhoea, malaria and leishmaniasis among those forced to abandon their homes by the war. They also remain the backbone of the 'People's Health Days' which have taken on added importance where regular health services have been disrupted due to the war.

Recent trends

New forms of community participation have emerged alongside the old. Every Saturday morning over 100 mothers in Ciudad Sandino now take part in health classes. The classes are organised by the women's organisation AMNLAE, the non-governmental agency CISAS, and the local health centre. On returning home, participants are able to pass on their knowledge to neighbours and friends. The emphasis is less on mobilising volunteers than on educating the community as a whole.[33]

The structures for participation are changing. The national level of the People's Health Council was abolished in 1986 because, as one MINSA leader put it, "It had become an empty, bureaucratic organisation with no particular function". In 1989 a new type of national council was established in order to promote the campaign to reduce infant and child mortality (see Chapter 9).

As the health system has been decentralised, community participation has been able to respond better to local conditions.[34] In Managua, for example, neighbourhood health commissions have been formed where high rates of clinic or hospital attendance are noted for preventable diseases. Doctors are sent to make door-to-door visits to identify cases. *Brigadistas* then take ongoing responsibility for up to 20 homes each in target areas.

Many people still become health volunteers. These *brigadistas* are now more often housewives and church activists than students. Their bravery and motivation seem endless. Jorge Rodriguez was a *brigadista* in the rural north. In January 1988 he was kidnapped by the *Contras* and has not been heard from since. His 19-year-old daughter Olivia completed her training in April to take his place. Asked why she would take on such a dangerous task, she replied, "For the health of Nicaragua's children and the memory of my father". An elderly rural birth attendant, when asked why she risked her life, replied, "Because I'm tired of seeing my children, and the children of this country, die of diarrhoea".

Community participation has become a major feature of the Nicaraguan health system. This enormous force has run up against serious political, financial, and administrative constraints. The resolution of these problems in the future will depend on evolving new forms of participation which place more power and initiative in the hands of the *brigadistas*.

Chapter 5: Mass Mobilisations

"We do not believe that health institutions will make people healthy. The protagonists of health are the people themselves."
(Dora Maria Tellez, Minister of Health)

Scene: the health centre in Ciudad Sandino, a township about ten kilometres outside Managua.[1]

Time: about 1:30 in the afternoon on a 'People's Health Day'. Nearly 150 children have been vaccinated since the health team arrived at 8 a.m. this morning. Now the pace has slackened. Most mothers are at home feeding or bathing their children, or rocking them to sleep in hammocks.

Jimena puts a vial of polio vaccine back into a thermos flask and sits down on an empty bench. On the far side of the room two other health volunteers have begun dancing to American pop music playing on the radio. Others are chatting with the nurses or tidying up after the hectic morning. Some of the *brigadistas* are medical students. A few are 15 or 16-year-old high school students. Others are housewives with part-time jobs. Jimena, who is responsible for organising this vaccination post, normally runs a refreshment stand from her home.

Five stocky, middle-aged women wearing frilly white aprons now file through the doorway. One carries a huge bowl of rice on her head, another a bowl of coleslaw and fried pork rind wrapped in banana leaves. A third brings a plastic bucket filled with a sugary fruit drink. The women immediately set about serving the *brigadistas* and nurses, laughing and joking with them as they eat. When Jimena and the others have finished, the women move on to the next vaccination post at the local primary school.

At about 3:00 p.m. a dozen children take to the streets, banging pots and pans and yelling:

"Parents! Bring in your children to be vaccinated! We don't want any cases of polio in our barrio! Vaccinate them! Every child deserves to grow up healthy!"

A few stragglers arrive, but Jimena's records show that two babies from the neighbourhood have still not been brought in. She sends off two *brigadistas* to vaccinate them at home.

Finally, around 5 p.m., Jimena checks her records for the last time: every baby and young child in the neighbourhood is now up-to-date with its measles and polio vaccinations. She picks up a megaphone and goes out into the muddy streets, shouting:

"It has just been learned that Block 8 has been liberated from the scourges of polio and measles. The children are victorious!"

Eradicating polio

Three times a year, between January and March, some 20,000 *brigadistas* immunise children in health posts, community centres, schools and homes. Before 1979 immunisation coverage was pitifully low. Fewer than 5% of young children were immunised against diseases such as measles, polio, tetanus, whooping cough, diphtheria and tuberculosis.[2] Sporadic campaigns led by First Lady Hope Somoza left the great majority of children unprotected against these diseases, which killed hundreds of children each year and left many more disabled.

In late 1979 a series of epidemics swept the country: first polio, then measles, and finally whooping cough. Doctors and nurses responded by organising weekend trips to immunise children in rural areas, where they met with some resistance. People opposed to the Sandinistas and their health initiatives (including some doctors) spread scare stories about the harmful effects of immunisation. A particularly imaginative tale was that the fluids for injection were not vaccines at all but Fidel Castro's urine. Most doctors resented what they saw as an incursion onto their 'turf'. "I won't say anything now," said one, "but these people have no right to come into this neighbourhood and interfere. They think medicine is all politics. But what will they do when they get sick once they have destroyed the medical profession and there are no more doctors?"

In any case, weekend trips by volunteers would not succeed in immunising more than a small minority of young children. Nor would the formal health system, with its limited personnel and facilities, be able rapidly to accelerate immunisation coverage. A new way had to be found to make immunisations more accessible and to persuade parents to take advantage of them.

It was the Literacy Campaign of 1980 which showed the way forward. In some areas, literacy volunteers had started polio immunisation campaigns. The oral polio vaccine was cheap, safe and easy to use: volunteers could easily be trained to administer two drops into a child's mouth. Mexico and Brazil had already followed Cuba's example of organising polio vaccination campaigns involving tens of thousands of volunteers.[3] In late 1980 MINSA decided to organise a national polio vaccination campaign during the first few months of 1981.

The campaign would consist of six steps. First, volunteers would be recruited by community organisations and trained in a one-day workshop. Second, volunteers would make a census of all families in their area to identify children who should be vaccinated and to explain to parents why vaccination was important. Third, national publicity would blanket the country with information just prior to and during the campaign day. Fourth, on a 'People's Health Day', volunteers would set up temporary vaccination posts in community centres, schools, health posts, or private homes (one post for every 100-200 residents) and vaccinate as many children as possible. Fifth, within three days they would carry out a 'clean-up' campaign, going from house to house to vaccinate children not brought to the vaccination post. Finally, they would fill in reporting forms which showed how many children in need of vaccination had been covered and how many were still unvaccinated.

The plan seemed to make sense, but would it work? Would there be enough volunteers, and would they be able to vaccinate correctly? Would supplies of vaccines be adequate? And would parents be sufficiently motivated to bring their children to the vaccination posts? There was no way of knowing in advance.

The 1981 campaign turned out to be highly successful. Estimated coverage with oral polio vaccine rose from about 24% to 70% among all under-one-year-olds.[5] The campaign also made apparent many weaknesses in the system. In the south, there were insufficient volunteers

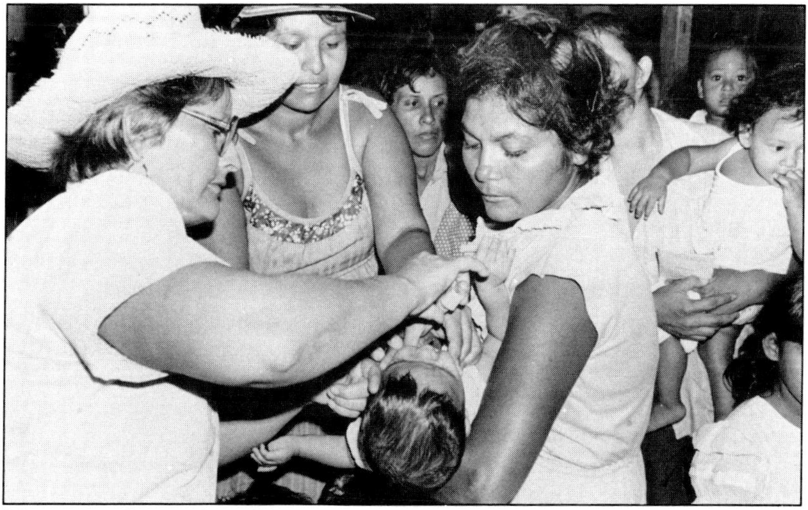

BARRICADA

Mothers bring their children to a health centre for polio vaccination on a 'People's Health Day'.

Fig. 5.1

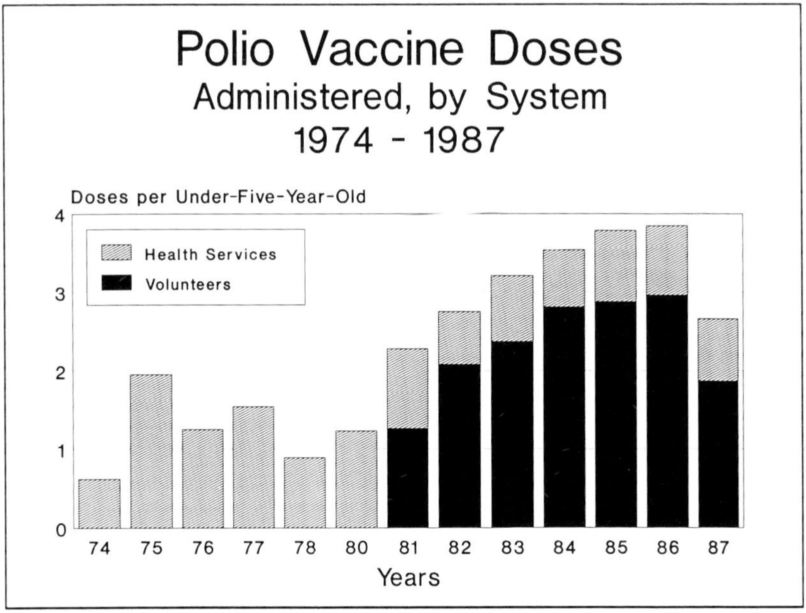

During the early 1980s the total number of polio vaccine doses administered exceeded the number actually needed. This 'overkill' helped to ensure adequate population coverage. While the health care system continued to administer vaccines, the increase in doses was due to the activities of volunteers in health campaigns.

and large numbers of children went unvaccinated. In the north there were enough volunteers, but many parents failed to bring their children to vaccination posts because they had not been properly informed about the benefits and safety of immunisation. Many volunteers lacked the training or maturity to carry out their tasks effectively: census information, for example, was often incomplete or inaccurate. There were also logistical problems: in many places the amount of vaccine available was insufficient; in other areas there was not enough 'cold chain' equipment.

In hundreds of meetings throughout the country, health workers and community leaders met to evaluate the 1981 campaign and plan the campaign for 1982. Health education activities were stepped up, volunteers were retrained, regular health workers were trained, and logistical systems were improved. The results in 1982 were even better, and by 1983 the system was running even more successfully than anyone had dared imagine. Polio coverage reached 80% of children under five, with most doses being given on the three People's Health Days between January and March (see Figure 5.1).

Fig. 5.2

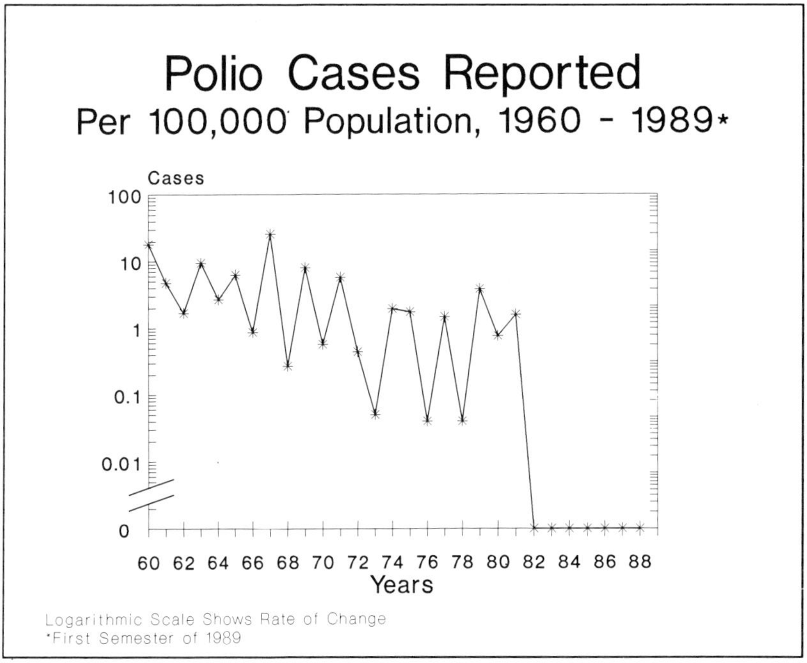

Reporting from past decades, though incomplete, shows a slow decline in the number of cases reported. From 1982 to 1988, no new polio cases were reported.

Even more important, the campaigns were being planned and implemented by People's Health Councils with only technical assistance from the Ministry of Health (MINSA). By 1983 most parents understood the importance of immunisation against polio, and wanted it for their children. "We don't see immunisation campaigns as a medical question," said Lea Guido, then Health Minister, "but as a demand which comes from the people." No cases of polio were reported in Nicaragua between 1982 and 1988, (see Figure 5.2).

Broadening the campaign

Enthusiasm for this approach to polio prevention was so great that, in 1981, MINSA administered measles and diphtheria-pertussis-tetanus (DPT) immunisations on People's Health Days. Since new skills were needed to administer these injectable vaccines, volunteers were given additional training.[6] Health educational activities within the community, however, were sadly lacking. As a result, many parents objected to their children being vaccinated against two or three diseases in a single session.

Fig. 5.3

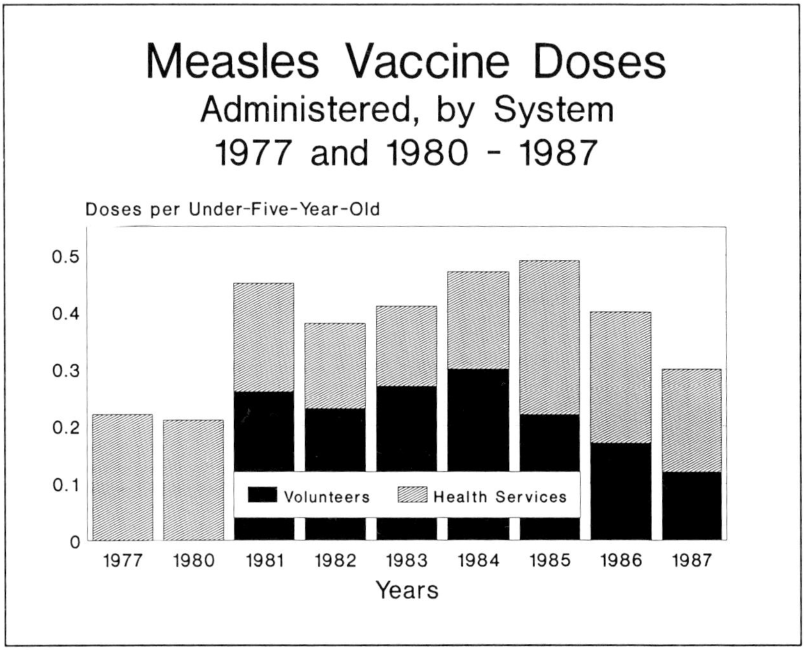

Although the number of doses of measles vaccine doubled after the revolution, coverage was still inadequate. The rise in doses administered is due both to the health care system and the activities of volunteers.

Waiting times at vaccination posts were also longer because of the greatly increased workload on volunteers and staff. Even with these limitations, measles coverage doubled to 40%,[7] with volunteers providing 55% of all vaccine doses (see Figure 5.3).

DPT coverage also increased, but only to a level of 22% coverage. In 1982 DPT was dropped from the campaign as it was thought that clinics and health posts could do the job better. Continuing low levels of DPT coverage led to its reintroduction in the 1986 immunisation campaign.

Measles coverage rose to 58% in 1985 but fell off in 1987. The proportion of all immunisations provided by campaigns also fell. This decline is related to the *Contra* war, because communities in areas under the threat of *Contra* attack were unable to organise effective health campaigns. Several years without access to vaccines created a large pool of vulnerable children. Under these conditions, one case of measles can lead to an epidemic.

Such an epidemic occurred in the war zones of Regions 1 and 6 in 1985 and 1986, where nearly 500 cases were reported. Special teams made emergency forays into the war zones to provide measles vaccine.

Fig. 5.4

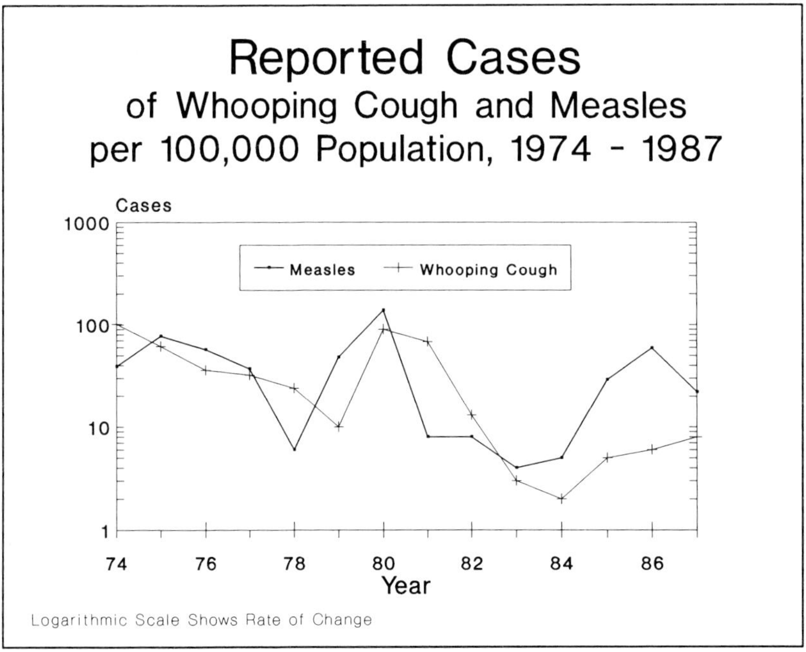

Epidemics of whooping cough and measles were noted in the year following the revolution. Levels then declined until 1985, when the higher number of cases in war zones plus improved reporting led to an increase in the reported cases of both these diseases.

By late 1986 the epidemic was brought under control. Greatly improved reporting of vaccine-preventable diseases helped control the epidemic, but makes direct comparisons with pre-revolutionary case-reporting data impossible (see Figure 5.4).

Numerous epidemics of vaccine-preventable diseases have prompted other Central American countries to organise community-based immunisation campaigns in recent years. In El Salvador a temporary truce, arranged three times a year through the good offices of the Catholic Church and the Red Cross, in the war between rebel forces and the Government allows health workers and volunteers to vaccinate throughout the country. National or localised immunisation campaigns are also organised in Honduras and Guatemala, but have not so far achieved the same degree of community involvement as in Nicaragua.

Mobilising against malaria

Malaria control was the only public health programme in Nicaragua which achieved significant coverage before 1979.[8] Funded by international donors in the 1950s, the programme consisted mainly of periodic pesticide sprayings in houses to kill the malaria-transmitting *Anopheline* mosquitoes. Communities were not actively involved in these activities, which were carried out by technicians with no relation to the rest of the health system. The initial results of the malaria control programme were dramatic. As in other countries, however, the mosquito's astonishing ability to develop resistance to new pesticides meant that large-scale outbreaks of the disease continued to be common.

Anti-malaria activities ground to a halt during the insurrection against Somoza. By July 1979 the malaria control system was in complete disarray and the number of cases reached epidemic levels not seen since anti-malaria campaigns began in the 1950s. As the demand for an effective response grew, the Government searched for solutions. Campaigns were organised to clean up places where mosquitoes bred, but these achieved little.

Health planners began to re-evaluate their strategy. Previous efforts had concentrated on attacking the mosquitoes to protect the people. But people were the only known reservoir for the disease. What would happen if they tried instead to eliminate the malaria parasites carried in the blood of infected people? If this were done on a wide enough scale, a whole generation of mosquitoes would live and die without becoming infected, thus breaking the chain of transmission.

An extremely ambitious plan was developed to administer anti-malarial drugs to the entire population above one year of age during three days in 1981. It would be a massive undertaking. Many thousands of volunteers would be needed to inform and motivate every family and to distribute the right quantities of tablets to every person in the country. Once again, the 'multiplier' strategy pioneered by the National Literacy Crusade provided the organisational basis.[9] A 'core' of 120 malaria health educators were trained. They each trained 10 volunteers as 'multipliers'.[10] These, in turn, trained and supervised a total of 73,000 health *brigadistas*, who were responsible for educating their own communities according to the guiding principle: "Only the people can educate the people".

In September, six weeks before the campaign began, community groups, government workers and school children began packing 35 million anti-malaria tablets into 9 million envelopes, colour-coded by dosage for different age groups. The national youth organisation conducted a door-to-door census, using each visit to explain the reasons for the campaign. More than 2,300,000 persons (87% of the country's estimated population) were registered in this way.

Every available means of communication was used to arouse public awareness and promote campaign messages. The country's three daily newspapers published about 300 advertisements, cartoons and articles explaining the purpose of the campaign and how it would be organised.

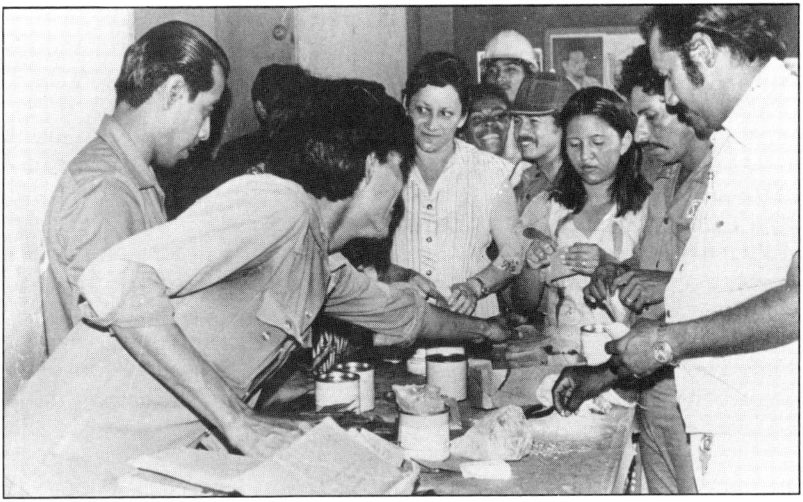

E BARRETO / BARRICADA

Volunteers pack antimalarial medicines for the nation-wide malaria campaign in 1981. A total of 9 million colour-coded envelopes were filled with appropriate dosages of tablets.

Television stations broadcast promotional 'spots'. Radio stations, asked to read campaign messages 12 times a day, responded by broadcasting them 20 or 30 times a day. Campaign posters were put up in thousands of public places, street theatre groups gave impromptu performances, and families hung home-made banners out of windows. Priests gave information about the campaign to their congregations. Volunteers made house-to-house visits, toured the streets making megaphone announcements, and gave talks at bonfire meetings, schools and work places.

This massive educational effort was in sharp contrast to the anti-malaria sprayings of the past, which had not attempted to involve the people in any active way. The independence of the malaria control system had long been accepted by doctors, who in any case had little interest in providing care in rural areas where malaria was common. But this massive campaign seemed a direct threat to doctors. It blanketed rural and urban areas alike, and focused on the distribution of pills rather than sprayings. It seemed to many physicians that this campaign was another attempt to weaken their social and political grip on society. Some doctors decided to strike back.

Physicians associated with opposition political parties published an article in *La Prensa* newspaper entitled (paradoxically) "Doctors Offer to Assist Campaign".[11] This article cited alleged cases of blindness, spontaneous abortion, amnesia and sudden death from chloroquine and primaquine — the two drugs to be used in the campaign.

Similar negative publicity was spread by an opposition radio station within the country and by anti-Sandinista radio stations broadcasting from neighbouring Honduras and Costa Rica. The anti-campaign messages claimed that anyone refusing to take the anti-malaria tablets would be fined, prevented from leaving the country, or refused medical treatment should they contract malaria. More fantastic still was the claim that the tablets were really brainwashing chemicals sent from Cuba and Russia in order to make the population communist. In addition, *Contras* threatened to kill volunteers and health workers — including the Pan American Health Organisation representative in Nicaragua — for promoting the campaign.

The Sandinistas contributed to the politicisation of the campaign. Some claimed (unrealistically) that the medicines used had no side effects. With US military manoeuvres starting on the Honduran side of the border, Nicaraguan military and political leaders were seen everywhere taking anti-malarial medicines and encouraging others to do so. Humberto Ortega, head of the armed forces, announced: "Taking the tablets to control malaria is key to our internal defence, just as the army protects us from the external aggressor."

Some Sandinista activists saw the anti-malaria campaign as a test of revolutionary faith, and the FSLN leadership had to quash an attempt to pass legislation which would have outlawed opposition to the campaign. In the end, the right of individuals to choose not to take part in the anti-malarial campaign was upheld.

In the final week of the campaign, a total of 240,000 health volunteers and helpers distributed anti-malaria tablets from house to house throughout the country. Tallies showed that more than 8 million doses of chloroquine and primaquine had been distributed to 1.9 million people — 70% of the total population.

During the next four months the number of confirmed cases of malaria dropped dramatically: the campaign is estimated to have prevented at least 9,200 new malaria cases.[12] But by March 1982, transmission of the *Plasmodium vivax* malaria parasite returned to the level of previous years. The more serious *Plasmodium falciparum* species was suppressed below expected levels for an additional three months.

The campaign did not succeed in eradicating malaria. It did, however, lay the basis for a new, more effective approach to combating malaria through community-based activities. It also succeeded in promoting widespread public awareness of malaria's symptoms and treatment. In addition, it created a new spirit of optimism and determination among community leaders and many thousands of new health volunteers.

It also succeeded in decentralising the Government's routine malaria control activities and in involving other government Ministries and community groups in the programme (see Figure 5.5). The new anti-malaria strategy now involves many health volunteers in seeking out

Fig. 5.5

Participants in the Antimalarial Campaign

- COMMUNITY GROUPS
  CDS - Block Associations
  AMNLAE - Women's Organisation
  JS - The Sandinista Youth Group
  MPS - The Civilian Defence Militia

- LABOUR ORGANISATIONS
  ATC - Rural Workers' Association
  CST - Federation of Sandinista Unions
  UNAG - Farmers' and Ranchers' Association
  ANDEN - Teachers' Union
  FETSALUD - Health Workers' Federation
  UNE - Office Workers' Union

- GOVERNMENTAL BODIES
  MINSA - Ministry of Health
  MED - Ministry of Education
  INRA - Ministry of Agriculture
  EPS - Army
  JRM - Municipal Governments
  MINCONS - Ministry of Construction
  INAA - Water Ministry
  IRENA - Natural Resources Ministry
  INTURISMO - Tourism Ministry

- OTHER GROUPS
  Christian and Other Religious Groups
  University and Other Student Groups

Source: Garfield R, Vermund SH, 'Health education and community participation in mass drug administration for malaria in Nicaragua', *Social Science and Medicine* 1986; 22 (8); 869-77.

cases of malaria, taking blood samples, making a speedy microscopic diagnosis, ensuring complete treatment of each proven case, and searching for further cases nearby. Under this strategy, the number of blood samples taken by health volunteers has doubled since 1981.[13]

The new approach has brought dramatic results. Between 1983 and 1985 the number of malaria cases diagnosed in areas not directly affected by the *Contra* war — and inhabited by just over half the total population

Fig. 5.6

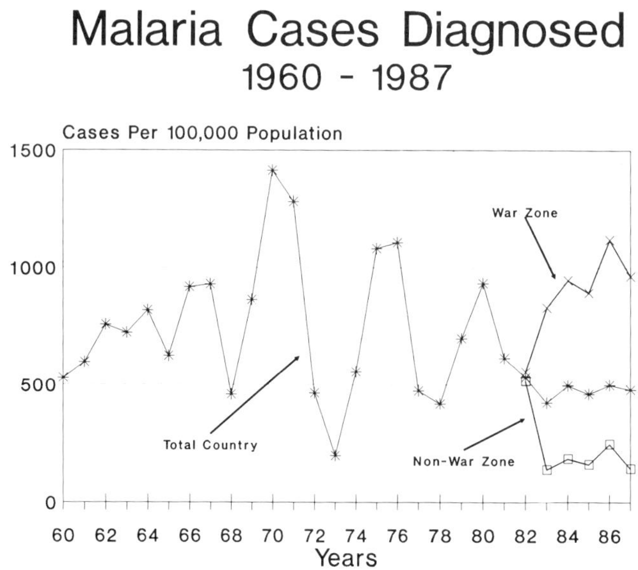

The incidence of malaria varied greatly from year to year in the decades prior to the revolution, largely because of changes in insecticides used. A more stable national rate since 1981 masks a marked divergence in incidence rates in the war and non-war zones of the country.

— dropped by 62%. An estimated 11,000 malaria cases were prevented between 1983 and 1986 in these areas. More importantly, the more serious *Plasmodium falciparum* species of malaria parasite dropped by 88%, nearly disappearing in the peaceful areas. Thus, for the first time, and almost without using pesticides, malaria was reduced to low levels in large parts of the country.[14]

In the war zones, where few malaria control activities can be safely maintained, thousands of people continue to suffer from this debilitating disease (see Figure 5.6). The proportion of all cases diagnosed in the war zones more than doubled between 1983 and 1986. The risk of malaria infection is now ten times greater in the war zone than in the rest of the country. Movements of refugees and *Contra* troops along the borders have also spread the disease in Honduras and Costa Rica.

How useful are mass mobilisations?

There is no doubt that the mass mobilisations against malaria and vaccine-preventable diseases gave a huge boost to efforts to control these

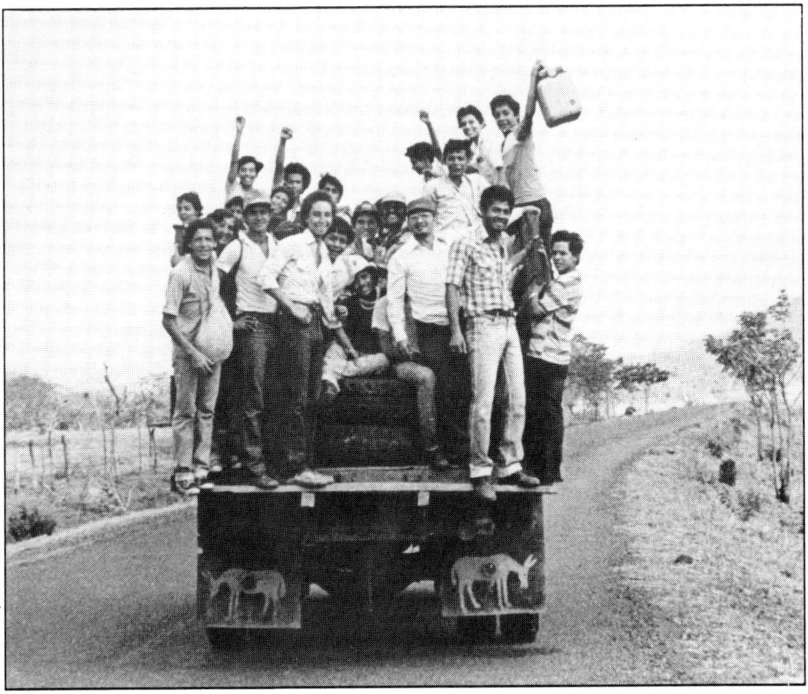

J ARAGON / BARRICADA

Volunteers set off for a day's vaccination campaign in Region 5, in 1983.

serious health threats. They also succeeded in involving large numbers of people in health activities. Other mass campaigns — such as those against dengue and rabies — also appear to have had an important impact and involved tens of thousands of volunteers.

But these mobilisations also have drawbacks. The first is their short-term, periodic nature, which relegates health education to a place of secondary importance. Another drawback is the shift away from routine, on-going health services that campaigns can cause.[15] According to Carolina Siu, formerly of the Division of Preventive Medicine:

"Mobilisations can raise our level of immunisation coverage rapidly, but they should not be idealised as the best solution. Many children are missed in these mobilisations or receive vaccines before or after the optimal age. Immunisation is only one component of the health needs of a child, and it should not be treated in isolation from the others. We must continue the campaigns to raise coverage right now, but in the long run our efforts to build up the basic health service system will be more important, and will do away with the need for some campaigns."

A third drawback of mass mobilisation is its tendency to alienate the medical profession. In the 1970s, doctors had become accustomed to lending their services on a charitable basis to short-term campaigns which did not involve the community in setting priorities or making decisions. The status and power of the medical profession was thus reinforced rather than threatened. Many Sandinista activists had something very different in mind. They viewed community mobilisations as a way of demonstrating how much ordinary citizens could achieve *without* the help of doctors.

This often meant bypassing the medical profession. Volunteers were trained to give polio and measles vaccinations, and community leaders took responsibility for organising People's Health Days. Oral rehydration posts were set up in community centres or private homes. These were important steps in giving ordinary people the skills and confidence to take greater initiative in health matters. But they were perceived by many doctors as a threat to their professional status and power. Some tried to obstruct these initiatives. Others simply ignored them or refused to cooperate with them. Community-led initiatives probably contributed to the decision of many doctors to leave the country (see Chapter 10).

The enormous power and importance of the medical profession cannot be ignored indefinitely. When organised medicine is openly hostile to the purposes or methods of mass health campaigns, passive or active sabotage is certain to follow, and society becomes more polarised. On the other hand, doctors have the potential to make a major contribution to the success of such campaigns. They can provide volunteers with technical advice and skills, supply medicines and equipment, and organise training and evaluation sessions. They are also highly influential members of the community: the advice they give can be a critical factor in the success or failure of a health campaign.

According to Carolina Siu, "Before, in order to bypass the doctors, we recreated vertical structures for health campaigns. What we need now is to foster an interdependence between doctors, community leaders and volunteers."

It is still an open question whether health education and mass campaigns have led to the 'empowerment' of ordinary people in giving them the ability to take greater control of their own health. 'People's Health Days' certainly succeeded in involving thousands of people in health activities. But repetition of the same slogans and activities often became more an act of political faith than a genuine liberating process. According to Dr. Leonel Arguello, Director of the Division of Preventive Medicine:

"To change someone's behaviour by concentrating efforts on one day can help. But what about next month or next year? We need to pay less attention to slogans and put more emphasis on reaching a basic understanding. Only then will the people be in a position to take the initiative, rather than just respond to MINSA requests."

Chapter 6: The War on Health

"Stop your medical work or we will burn the clinic and you with it."
(Note left by *Contra* troops for nurse in El Cedro, Region 6. Three weeks later, on 18 March 1988, the clinic was destroyed. The nurse fled to safety.)

Just before daybreak on the morning of 14 April 1984, Dr. Roberto Valle Gonzalez woke to the clatter of small arms fire and the crash of mortar shells. Rushing out of the flimsy wooden house adjoining the health centre, he flung himself into a shallow trench. Moments later a child, blood spurting from its mouth, fell into his arms. It was, he later recalled, "the worst moment I ever experienced as a doctor — watching that child die while I was helpless to act".

They were under attack by *Contras* — the army of peasants and former National Guardsmen organised by the US Central Intelligence Agency (CIA) to weaken and overthrow the Sandinista Government. Dr. Valle was marched away by *Contras*, leaving behind a shattered health centre and a burnt-out ambulance. The health centre, built only a year earlier, had been the first ever in Sumubila, a settlement in a remote area of the Atlantic Coast inhabited by the Sumu and Miskito peoples. Dr. Valle managed to escape 30 days later, and eventually found his way back to safety. Sumubila was left without a permanent health service until 1989.

Targeting the health system

Contra attacks on health and social services began soon after the Sandinistas came to power. During the National Literacy Crusade in 1980, bands of ex-National Guardsmen killed three young literacy volunteers near the Honduran border in the north of the country. In 1982, a nurse and two Cuban school teachers were murdered by counter-revolutionaries. Following preparations in Florida, *Contras* equipped and supplied from bases in Honduras infiltrated northern Nicaragua in 1983 while others crossed the border from Costa Rica in the south. By the end

Fig. 6.1

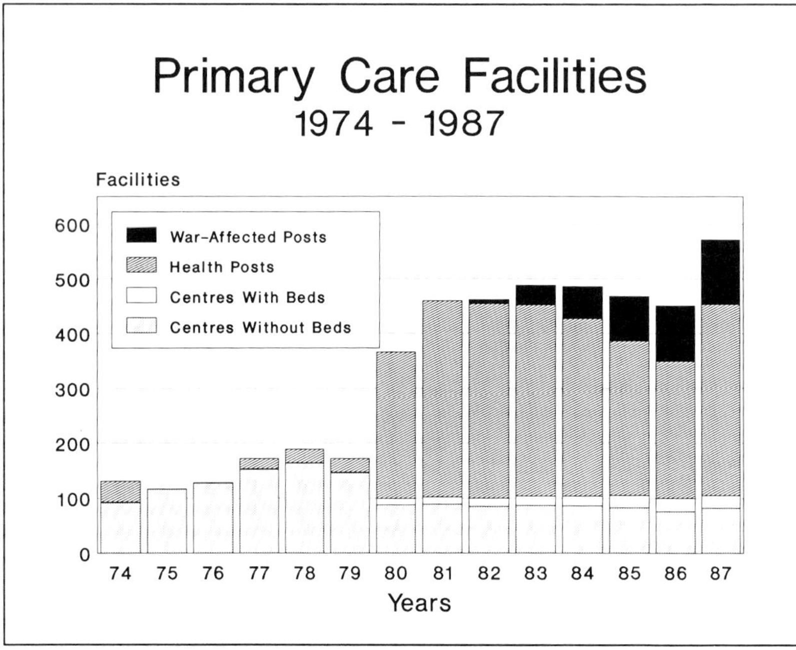

The rapid growth in health facilities in the early 1980s slowed down in the late 1980s due to the destruction or closing of health facilities in war-affected areas.

of 1983 *Contra* forces were estimated to number between 12,000 and 15,000 troops.

Health facilities have been among the *Contras*' prime targets.[1] By the end of 1987, 128 of the country's 600 health facilities had been destroyed, damaged or forced to close (see Figure 6.1). The losses included one hospital, seven health centres and 115 posts in six regions of the country. The construction of 22 others was abandoned because of the war.[2]

While attacks have taken place over a wide area, they have been especially intense in Regions 1 and 6, near the Honduran border in the north of the country. There were hopes that the *Contra* war would end after the five Central American Presidents signed a regional peace accord in Esquipulas, Guatemala, in August 1987. Attacks have decreased, but still continue. In the 12 months which followed the signing of the peace accord in Esquipulas, eight health workers were kidnapped, two wounded, and two killed in Region 6.[3] A Red Cross ambulance was one of three attacked in the region during the same period. This was the first attack on the Red Cross since those by the National Guard in 1979. Two health centres and two child-feeding centres were also attacked. Although such actions may continue in the future, their frequency is diminishing as the *Contra* army slowly disintegrates.

Contras target health services as part of the social infrastructure established by the Sandinista Government. Their forces have either destroyed or damaged 67 schools and 125 social service centres serving 17,000 children and elderly people.[4] Another 503 schools and 800 adult education centres have been closed due to threats of attack, and 170 adult education teachers have been killed. The Government also halted the building of 2,000 rural homes and abandoned the construction of rural roads, water supplies, and sanitation facilities. It was estimated that in rural areas about 45% of people were without adequate water and 85% lacked adequate sanitation facilities.[5]

By the end of 1985 close to 10% of the country's inhabitants and a quarter of those who lived in war zones — about 300,000 people — had lost access to health services because of the war.[6] Some facilities have been destroyed and rebuilt several times. The health centre in the township of Cerro Colorado, in Region 6, was blown up for the fourth time by *Contra* troops on 21 October 1987. Before leaving, they gathered the local people together and told them: "As often as you rebuild this clinic we will return to destroy it". It has not been rebuilt again.

In the small town of Mancotal, near the Honduran border, the health post was destroyed three times. On the first two occasions the people rebuilt it, despite *Contra* threats of reprisals. After the third burning, health activities were transferred to the homes of three local *brigadistas*. Each took charge of a portion of the medicines to limit the risk to any one of them. In late 1988 the people of Mancotal began to rebuild the health centre again.[7]

Contras also raid government health services and *brigadistas*' homes for medical supplies and equipment, especially in isolated rural areas. In the formerly neglected Atlantic Coast region, where many new health facilities have been built since 1979, *Contras* have robbed clinics at least 30 times since 1982. Dr. Domingo Vanegas was kidnapped from his social service post in South Zelaya and obliged to provide medical care to the *Contras* for almost a year:[8]

"If I was short of supplies to attend to the *Contra* sick and wounded they would take me to the houses of *brigadistas* and say 'Take what you want, take everything if you need it'. The only reason they didn't kill the *brigadistas* was because they were a source of medical supplies."

Deaths and injuries

The Nicaraguan Government reports a total of 6,760 people killed, more than 10,000 injured, and a total of 7,226 taken hostage or prisoner by *Contra* forces from 1982 to 1988[9] (see Figure 6.2). Almost 60% of the dead were civilians, including 455 children and 355 women (see Figure 6.3). This represents a death rate of 0.2%, more than ten times higher

Fig. 6.2

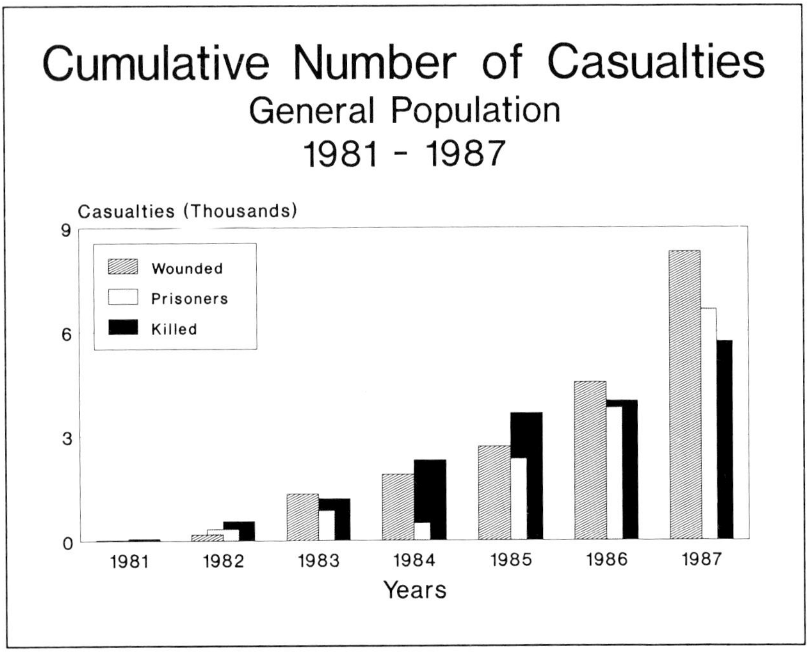

than the death rate experienced by the US population due to the Vietnam War.[10] It represents the equivalent of 500,000 deaths in the USA or 100,000 deaths in the UK. Less reliable estimates of *Contra* casualties suggest that close to 20,000 deaths have occurred among these forces.

Nearly one in every ten hospital admissions between 1983 and 1986 was for war-related injuries.[11] Among survivors of *Contra* attacks, the most serious wounds are to the lower limbs as a result of explosions caused by mines or mortars.[12] About half of those injured are civilians. A typical incident occurred on the road from Pantasma to Jinotega, in Region 6, on 20 October 1986, when a truck full of civilians hit a *Contra* land mine. The force of the blast blew out the entire back of the truck and killed four women, a seven-year-old girl and a man. Among the 43 injured survivors, six had amputations on the spot and five more had leg amputations within days.

Approximately 0.2% of the Nicaraguan population now has some kind of physical disability. About half of these 6,000 people were disabled in the *Contra* war. If the problem is not a leg or foot amputated in the war, it may be a missing hand or forearm from a home-made fragmentation bomb during the 1978-79 insurrection. Others have a deformity resulting from polio, or a spinal-cord injury from the 1972 earthquake. Treatment and rehabilitation for these people are a heavy burden on the country's

Fig. 6.3

Nicaraguans Directly Affected by the War, 1980 - 1987, in Government-Controlled Territory.

	Dead	Injured	Hostages, Prisoners
Total:	6760	10,546	7226
Of Which:			
Under 15 years:	455	1542	691
15-20 years:	1098	1865	1545
Male:	6405	8943	6363
Female:	355	1603	863
Military:	2961	8507	1060
Peasants:	2311	1657	5701
Professional, Technical, Workers, or Students:	1488	382	465
Of Which,			
Health Workers:	48	26	32
Of Which,			
Doctors	25	18	17
Nurses	9	7	6

Source: INSSBI

already over-stretched medical and social welfare services.[13]

Many war deaths are a consequence of limitations in health services caused by the war itself. On the night of 2 July 1987, US doctors Susan Cookson and Tim Takaro were woken up when a wounded government soldier was brought to their poorly equipped health post near Matagalpa. Initially it seemed that the young man had only a gunshot wound to the knee, but they soon realised that he had abdominal injuries and was haemorrhaging. Hospital surgery was needed, but the army could not risk making the journey at night because of the threat of *Contra* attack. "Our

Fig. 6.4

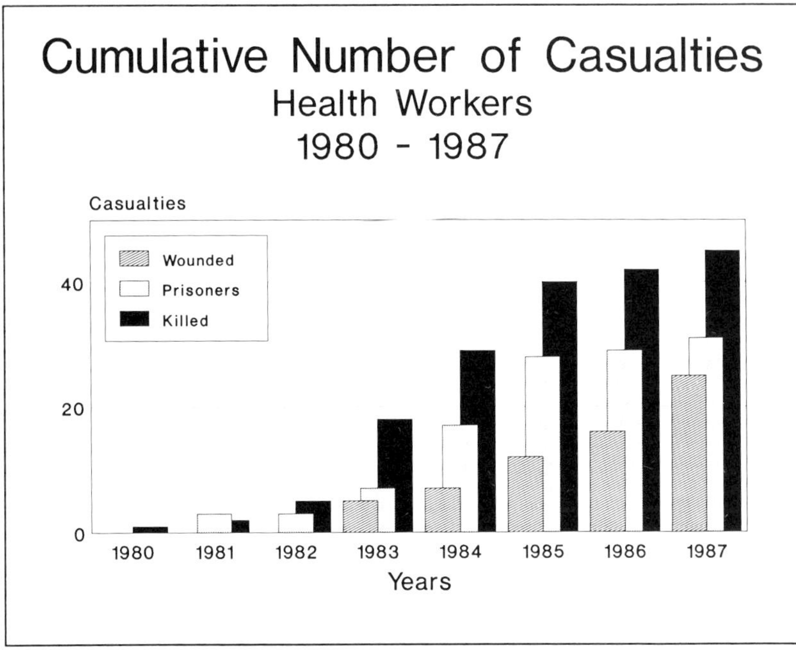

job," Dr. Cookson later recalled, "became a race against time and the haemorrhage to keep him alive until daybreak. The race was lost at 2:38 a.m."

Attacks on Health Workers

By December 1987, a total of 48 health workers, including 25 doctors and 9 nurses, had been killed by *Contras* (see Figure 6.4). Another 32 had been kidnapped and 26 wounded.[14] Some of those kidnapped, including Dr. Gustavo Sequiera, Vice-Dean of the Managua Medical School, and Dr. Myrna Cunningham, now Governor of Northern Zelaya province, were high-ranking medical leaders. Most victims, however, were young nurses and doctors working in isolated rural communities.

In some cases, health workers were targeted and murdered while carrying out their professional duties. Such an attack claimed the lives of nurse Juana Cruz Padilla and ambulance driver Ambrosio Raudales Lopez, on 28 March 1983, as they were taking a patient by ambulance to Ocotal hospital. Both were tortured before being killed.

Other health workers have been killed when caught in an area under *Contra* attack. French physician Pierre Grosjean received a fatal shrapnel wound on 26 March 1983, during an attack on a village near Matagalpa where he was engaged in tropical medicine research. Nurse Marilu Reyes died in a *Contra* ambush in El Cua on 3 November 1984, when returning home after voting in the country's presidential election.

Brigadistas in the firing line

Nestor Castilblanco, a health *brigadista* in Region 6, was abducted from his home in August 1986. He had already been kidnapped by *Contras* three times before, and was warned each time not to take part in vaccination campaigns. This time they took him and three other male relatives. As his wife tried to follow, he yelled back: "I'm a dead man..." Next morning a search party found all four bodies, their eyes gouged out and testicles cut off.

The war has taken a heavy toll on the activities of health volunteers.[15] More than 40 have been killed and many more kidnapped. Hundreds have stopped volunteering because of death threats from *Contras*. Mary Elsberg, a health educator in South Zelaya, reported that the number of active *brigadistas* fell from 250 in 1983 to 60 in 1984. In 1986, when *Contra* activities lessened, the number of *brigadistas* in the area increased to 120. Dr. Tim Takaro works with health volunteers near the Honduran border: "Their number one fear is being killed or kidnapped by *Contras*. They try to keep good relations with both sides. I would say they are Sandinistas in one way or another. They see that the children now get medicine. They own the land they used to work for someone else. They see and want to participate in the progress."

Health campaigns and educational activities in the war zones have suffered from the threats, killings and destruction wreaked by counter-revolutionaries. Yet in many areas, despite a constant *Contra* presence, the Government's health initiatives are carried out by health volunteers. In order to avoid attracting the attention of the *Contra*, health campaigns in war zones are often held prior to or following their announced national date. In some areas, vaccination campaigns are held on a house-to-house basis so that families do not have to leave the relative safety of their homes.

The Health Ministry (MINSA) trains *brigadistas* for the armed forces, and armed guards sometimes accompany volunteers in dangerous areas. Initiatives to reach the people cut off by the war come not only from the Government. In some areas, progressive priests give *brigadistas* church identification cards. This is believed to confer some protection on the volunteer if he or she is kidnapped.

The *Contras* see health volunteers as representatives of the Sandinista Government. Dr. Manuel Alzugarey, a Cuban exile, is in charge of the Miami-based *Contra* medical organisation:[16]

"The *brigadistas* are working with the enemy. They are a legitimate target. These people should not be in the war zones. The Sandinistas are using them for propaganda... It's hard to instruct our troops on Geneva Convention rules when they don't even know where Geneva is."

Fig. 6.5

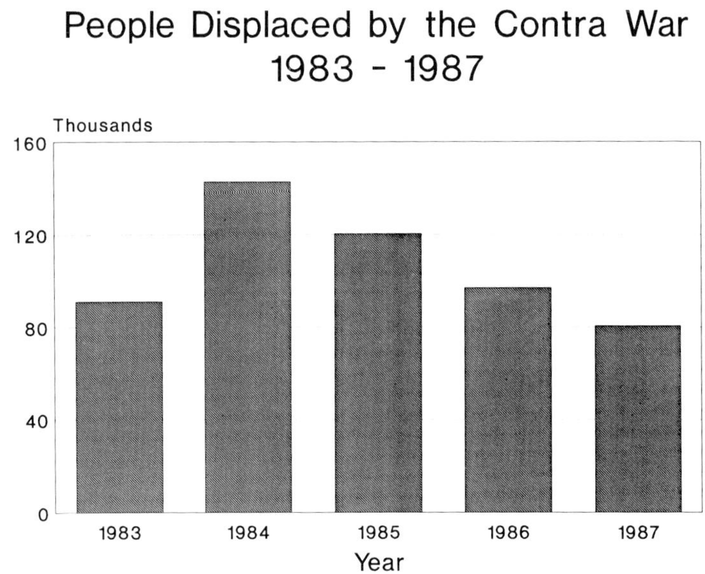

Although the largest group of people to flee their homes because of the *Contra* war did so in 1984, many more were displaced in the years which followed.

War-related diseases

Contra attacks, lack of basic supplies and disruption of food production have forced about 300,000 Nicaraguans to move from their homes (see Figure 6.5). Most have fled to Managua and other urban areas, placing a severe strain on the already inadequate social and economic infrastructure. At least 100,000 have settled in 145 new settlements established by the Government in areas near their original homes.[17] A health clinic and a school are among the first buildings to be constructed in these new communities. Water supplies, sanitation, and food production invariably lag behind.

In the cities, slum neighbourhoods (called 'spontaneous' or 'clandestine' settlements) seem to appear overnight. These neighbourhoods have no lights, running water, or sewers. The Epidemiology Department of the regional MINSA office is responsible for identifying, visiting, assisting, and monitoring the health of people in these settlements. In 1988, 44 of them were classified as unhealthy and 19 as extremely dangerous.

These large-scale population movements — coupled with the

inaccessibility of large areas due to *Contra* attacks — have led to an upsurge in epidemics. The most serious and widespread of these is malaria. In the areas most seriously affected by the war, malaria control activities have been severely hampered. Malaria workers are reluctant to go into many areas, and visit war zones only briefly for cursory inspections. Regions 2 and 6 — both war- affected areas — reported 70% of all malaria cases in 1986, compared with only 35% in 1983. Before the war, the risk of contracting malaria was almost equal in what were to become the war and non-war zones. In the late 1980s, the risk was ten times greater in war zones.[18] The worst malaria situation is to be found in new settlements, where poor housing, stagnant water and over-crowding sometimes result in infection rates close to 100%.

Since 1983, some rural regions have became inaccessible to immunisation teams because of *Contra* activity. This break-down in immunisation coverage led to epidemics in those areas. In 1985-86, the first measles epidemic since 1979 affected several thousand children. The great majority of cases appeared in Regions 1 and 6, the two regions most affected by the *Contra* war (see Figure 6.6). In the department of Matagalpa, for example, the number of measles cases rose from 153 in 1985 to 956 in 1986.

There have also been smaller, localised epidemics. In early 1987, for example, Drs. Cookson and Takaro diagnosed six cases of meningococcal meningitis in Jinotega. Four cases were from Abisinia, a Miskito area in a nearby war zone. Under normal conditions health workers would have rushed to the area with antibiotics to treat the infected and halt the spread

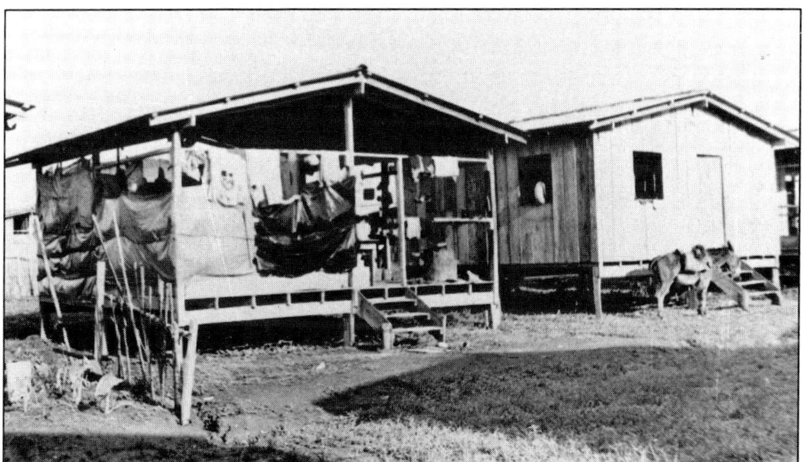

EL NUEVO DIARIO

Over 100,000 people have been housed in resettlement camps after being forced to flee from their homes because of the *Contra* war. Houses built at a new settlement, La Esperanza, by refugees.

Fig. 6.6

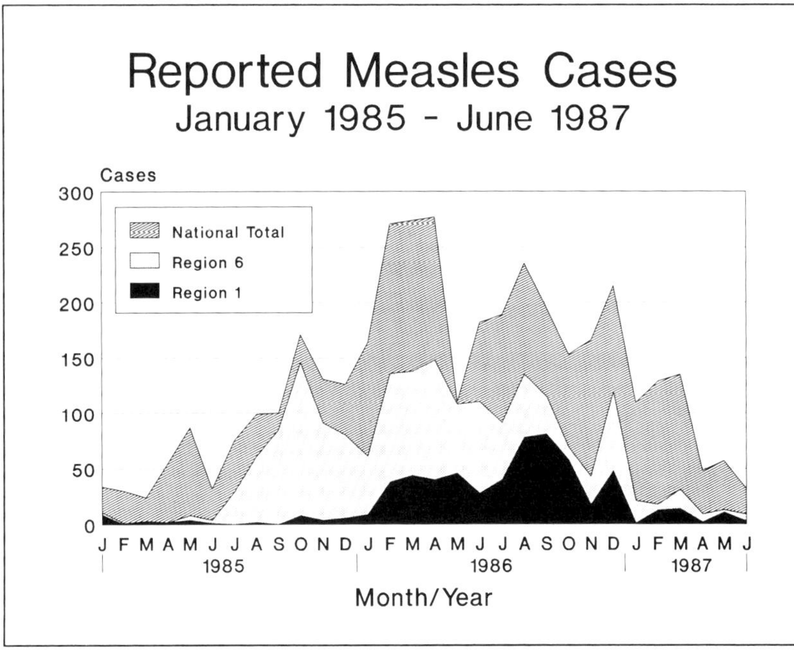

In the middle of 1985 a rapid rise in reported measles cases occurred in Region 6. The epidemic soon spread to Region 1. These two regions account for most reported measles cases during 1985 and 1986.

Source: Vigilancia Epidemiologica, MINSA.

of the disease. Since health workers could not safely enter the area, however, the disease rapidly assumed epidemic proportions and lasted for several months. "The sick here," said Cookson, "are war victims whose numbers are not reflected in government casualty figures."

The war is also a major cause of malnutrition, due to the disruption of planting and harvesting and the difficulty of ensuring a regular supply of supplementary foods to new settlements.[19] Malnutrition and the war caused the death of two-year-old Gloria Rosales, daughter of *brigadista* Pablo Rosales, who was killed by *Contras* (along with US volunteer Ben Linder) in 1987. After Pablo's death, the family's plantings and income declined, reducing their food supply. Within six months Gloria died, her body weakened by repeated bouts of diarrhoea and insufficient food.

According to Matagalpa nutritionist Ana Julia Gutierrez, import restrictions caused by credit shortages meant that in 1985 only about 20% of the children selected for a food supplementation programme in the region actually received food. The problem was exacerbated by a delay of several months in the arrival of foodstuffs caused by the mining of Nicaraguan ports by CIA operatives in 1984.[20]

Psychological effects

The psychological impact of the *Contra* war is the most difficult effect to quantify but may be the most far-reaching.[21] It affects three broad groups:

First are civilians living in war zones. Adults who see the results of *Contra* attacks on repeated occasions often wonder when death, torture or injury may catch up with them or their loved ones. They tend to be preoccupied with the present and experience psychological problems stemming from a sense of insecurity and vulnerability.

The second group consists of civilians who live and work outside the war zones. They do not see the violence, but hear about it from friends, relatives, at meetings, or via the news media. They often feel guilty about the immense sacrifices made by those in the war zones and feel helpless and depressed about their inability to do anything to change the situation.

The third group consists of military personnel, including conscripts and militia, both in and outside the war zones. They experience the same problems as other soldiers who do not know when or where they will next have to place their lives at risk. Nor — despite the concerted international efforts in 1987-89 to achieve peace — are they able to foresee an end to the hostilities. Battle psychosis, paranoid behaviour and depression are common.

Children living in war zones are particularly vulnerable to psychological trauma as a result of the war. In May 1988 a Needs Assessment Team from CARE estimated that 40,000-50,000 Nicaraguan children suffered some degree of trauma.[22]

A museum in the town of Esteli exhibits children's art. Such art can reveal children's feelings, preoccupations, and inner thoughts. Common themes in this exhibition included fear, loss and insecurity and the symbols in the drawings reflect the experience of the individual child. Asked to draw whatever she liked, 12-year-old Marbelli Palacios Blandon had drawn a house with many people, small and large, going in and out. In the doorway there was a coffin, and in other parts of the picture there were drawings of a garden, some flowers, and a heart. The child explained:

"They took my Daddy, dragged him away and killed him. Also, I painted the garden where we played with my Dad." Around the heart was written: "My heart is not quiet because they tortured my Daddy." And on one side: "This is my community, my Daddy they took away, dragged him, but I cried, screamed, and I want peace to come. Goodbye Daddy, I said while crying."

The psychological effects of war are more pervasive than this brief account can suggest. Terror invoked by sporadic death and destruction devastates one's sense of autonomy. US doctor Antonio Dager reflected,

"It is so easy to forget the attrition factor when war is looked at from a distance. Every time the lights went out, every time an extra shift of guard duty had to be done, every additional queue that wasted time sapping people's energy and morale, made them less able to rebuild the country. For the civilians, it was the sense of impotence, of waiting to see where the *Contras* would strike next, that was so demoralising."

Grief can also become overwhelming. Dr. Dager observed that many of the patients at Somoto hospital, just outside the war zone, were relatives of fallen soldiers. "Their grief kept them from eating, so they were brought in for intravenous fluids. One grandmother especially broke my heart. She was 85, all wrinkles, and repeated with her raspy voice 'Why couldn't I have died instead?' I tried everything: vitamins, saline, pep talks, and placebos, but nothing worked. By her fifth visit I wanted to escape out the back window rather than face the depth of her sadness again. My books say there is a natural limit to grief, but what do American psychiatrists know about the effects of interminable war?"

Effects of the embargo and financial boycott

Claiming Nicaragua to be a "serious and immediate threat to the security of the United States", the Reagan administration imposed an economic embargo in 1985. The war and economic embargo have caused serious shortages of essential drugs, medical supplies and surgical equipment. In early 1984, for example, a shipment of raw materials to produce drugs was delayed for three months due to the mining of Nicaragua's ports and patrols by US gunboats. Lack of reagents has led to cutbacks in the number of laboratory tests and X-rays provided by the health services.

More insidiously, basic materials needed for medical education, training and health programmes are in short supply. Paper shortages mean that medical students cannot copy their class notes to make up for the medical books which are unavailable. Shortages of pens, magic markers, slide projectors and posterboard have restricted health education activities. Journals, medical texts, and spare parts for equipment are in critically short supply.

Lack of finance means fewer scholarships in the medical and allied health training schools. The economic downturn and the war have led many health professionals to leave the country or seek private practice rather than government service. From 1984 to 1987 about a quarter of all MINSA employees left their posts each year, making continuity of programmes impossible. In these and similar ways, the war is felt every day throughout the country.

Low intensity warfare

In military terms, the *Contra* war is of 'low intensity'.[23] This is reflected in a comparison between 6,760 deaths among Nicaraguans in this war and 35,000 deaths during the insurrection of 1978-79. But damage to the

Fig. 6.7

Low-Intensity Wars in the 1980s
A Comparison of Nicaragua and Mozambique

	Nicaragua	Mozambique
Health Workers Killed	48	21
Taken Prisoner	32	45
Ambulances Destroyed	10	20
Health Posts Attacked or Closed	131 (22% of all)	484 (25% of all)
Destruction of Health Facilities (Millions)	$6	$20
Health as % of All Destruction	3%	4%

Source: Cliff J, Noormahomed AR, 'Health as a target: South Africa's destabilisation of Mozambique', *Social Science and Medicine* 1988: 27(7): 717-22.

country's social and economic infrastructure has been devastating. Living standards and the quality of services have declined sharply since the war intensified in 1983. It is estimated that more than three billion dollars' worth of damage has been done.[24] This is the result of a US policy aimed at undermining the Government rather than confronting it in conventional, land-based territorial warfare. The same tactic was used by rebel forces during the 1980s in 'low intensity' wars against progressive regimes in Angola and Mozambique.[25] (see Figure 6.7)

Low intensity warfare, according to Colonel John Waghelstein of US Army Special Forces, is "total war at the grassroots level", involving "political, economic and psychological warfare, with the military being a distant fourth".[26] The US objective is not to defeat the Sandinistas militarily, but to bring about their political downfall. Said Manuel Rodriguez, head of civil defence in the Ministry of Health: "They want to show that the Government cannot provide services". Zeno Bisoffi, an Italian doctor working in the north of the country, described the *Contras*' motivation in this way:

"Some of them lost power or money with the advent of the revolution. They want to come back to their areas and punish their neighbours for the improvements these people now enjoy. Others want to deny social benefits to the population because services increase the population's support for the Sandinistas. Somehow, they seem to feel that they can terrorise the peasants into passive submission, like in the old days of Somoza's rule."

The protagonists of low intensity warfare use disease as a political metaphor. The Reagan administration repeatedly referred to Nicaragua as a 'virus' or 'cancer' which had to be surgically removed.[27] Former White House spokesperson Patrick Buchanan called Nicaragua a 'malignant tumour' threatening the health of the whole Western Hemisphere: "There can be no negotiating with a cancer. Surgically precise military strikes are the necessary remedy."

The *Contras* do not fit a 'classical' model of a guerrilla army.[28] Rebel forces fighting wars of national liberation in countries such as Angola, Mozambique and Zimbabwe enjoyed the support of the majority of the population. They attacked government forces by surprise but usually left the local civilian population in peace. They had a broad, coherent political programme. The *Contras*, by contrast, have little support in Nicaragua. They attack civilian targets and avoid engagements with the Sandinista armed forces.[29] Their political agenda involves little more than trying to return to the pre-revolutionary status quo.

The Government's response

Three programmes involving health volunteers were mounted to mitigate some of the most harmful effects of the war. The first, a first-aid training programme, prepared 25,000 volunteers in wound management, resuscitation, evacuation of the injured and patient assessment. The second, which involves building 'refuges' to protect civilians from attack, comes from the experience of the FSLN during the insurrection of 1978-79. (A 'refuge' consists of a hole dug about five feet deep and covered with logs and earth to provide protection against bomb and mortar attacks.) Finally, fire control education and practice sessions are held periodically throughout the country to train people in responding to sabotage attacks. This training helped to reduce damage and speed up the evacuation of civilians following the *Contra* attack on petroleum storage tanks in Corinto in October 1983.

Paradoxically, the war has also led to some positive changes in the health system. Among these are more efficient use of resources, better organisation, the setting of clear priorities, and increased administrative decentralisation.[30] According to Health Minister Dora Maria Tellez: "The tighter things are, the better we have to organise things so as to obtain maximum usage of our resources." While concentrating formerly scattered rural communities into new settlements quickly led to localised epidemics, it has also made it much easier for health workers to reach families with preventive and curative services.

But the war has also distorted the way in which health and social

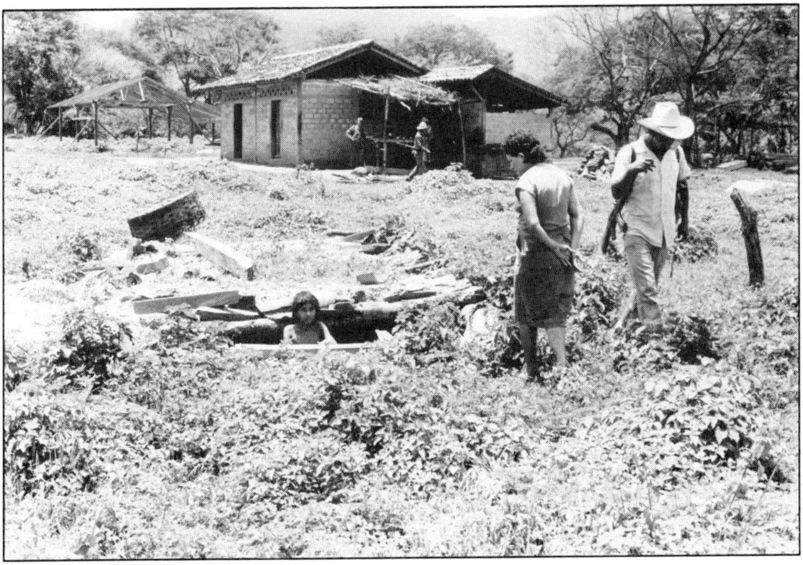

Santiago Arauz Cooperative, near the Honduran border, was attacked by *Contras* on 31 December 1984 and six people were killed. Several women and children took refuge in this shelter.

services have developed. When the *Contras* started losing the war in 1986, they laid many land mines to cover their retreat. This resulted, late in the war, in a rise in the number of amputations performed in Managua hospitals and a rapid rise in the number of permanently disabled citizens (see Figure 6.8). The Government has been forced to invest heavily in rehabilitation instead of other health programmes. Similarly, social welfare is focused on the 10,000 orphans resulting from the war, neglecting other children in need of care.

The deaths of a French and a German physician early in 1983 brought a sobering reassessment of the roles of foreign health workers in primary health care. Responding to the concerns of Western European Governments, MINSA moved foreign health workers from areas with frequent *Contra* activity to safer places. In 1986 foreigners were further restricted to living and working only in the capital cities of regions with frequent military activity. This caused many rural health and development projects to come to a halt and meant that the only foreign doctors who could still work in the war zones were from Cuba and the US.

In many rural areas the Government also halted construction of health facilities because of the war. Nevertheless, many new hospitals, health centres and health posts have been built in the war zones. These facilities, usually located in areas close to main roads and therefore more

Fig. 6.8

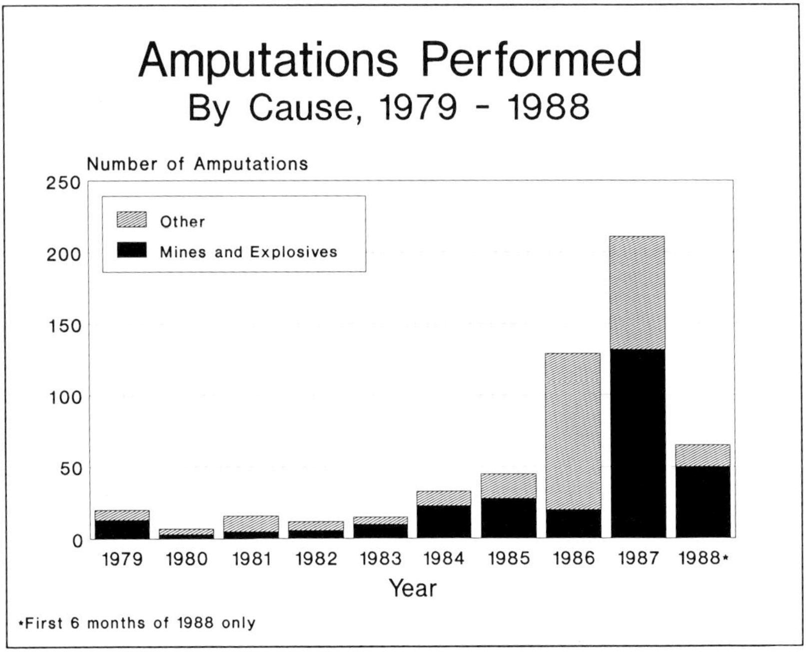

A shift in military tactics to hit-and-run attacks and the widespread use of mines toward the end of the *Contra* war was associated with a dramatic increase in the number of amputations carried out in Managua hospitals.

defensible, now form the backbone of the new health system in these areas. In the town of Jalapa, for example, only five miles from the Honduran border and twice put under siege by the *Contras*, new operating theatres were added to the government hospital in 1986, making it a more independent regional centre.

Hospitals in border regions function on a war footing.[31] The hospital in La Trinidad, near Esteli, for example, has become exclusively surgical, serving as the main treatment centre for war-related injuries in the north. A new surgical Army hospital has also been built at Apanas, in the north. In other hospitals in the north, up to 25% of all patients suffer from war-related injuries. These hospitals maintain empty beds in order to receive the war-injured at short notice. Even the major hospitals in Managua have contingency plans to handle up to three times their usual number of patients if necessary.

In the war zones Army doctors treat large numbers of civilian patients in order to fill the gap left by the destruction or closure of health centres and posts. This has been made possible through the recruitment of more physicians into the Army, the mobilisation of civilian doctors (see Figure

Fig. 6.9

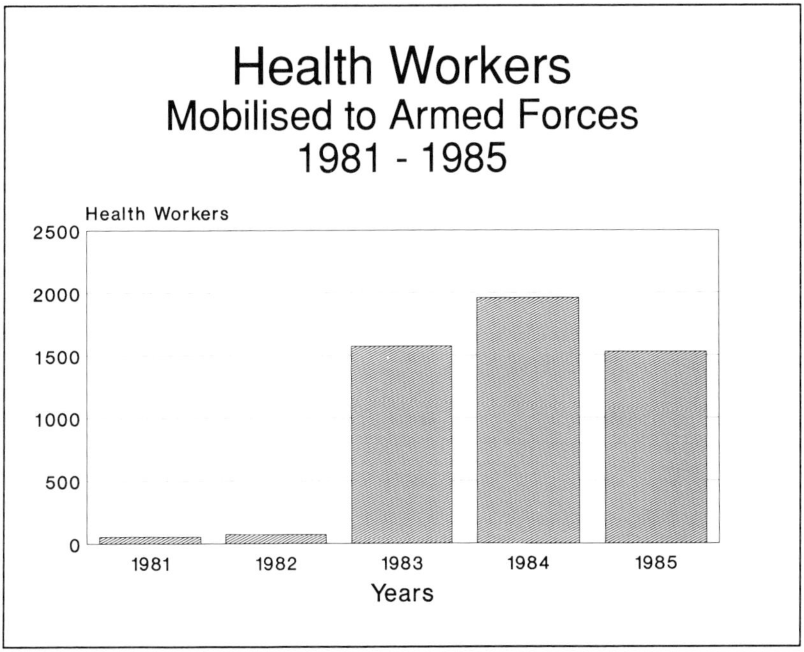

Many civilian health workers were mobilised to support the army in the early years of the *Contra* war.

6.9), the creation of teams of medical students in health brigades for three to eight months' stints, and close coordination between the civilian and military medical authorities in the war zones.

Health as a bridge to peace

In May 1988, 500 health workers took advantage of a 60-day cease-fire to re-establish contact with people in areas controlled by the *Contras* near the Honduran border. They started to enter the war zone in March, before the cease-fire, under the protection of the Red Cross and the Catholic Church. In May they fanned out across a vast area in pairs. In most communities the presence of health workers was welcome. The teams' goal was to learn what were the greatest health needs after five years of isolation. Dr. Alvaro Ramirez, who organised the teams, saw this as a chance to rebuild. He said, "When peace comes, MINSA will be a purely social institution, so we are trying to get a new image now. We want to talk less about the revolution and do more for it."[32] Dr. Amado Gavidia, a team leader, added, "We must think about building health for the future, because we are not always going to live at war."

Predictably, they found a population that was sicker and poorer than in other rural areas. Only six percent of the people had latrines, 70% of children were malnourished, and 80% of pregnant women were at high risk of poor birth outcomes. Tuberculosis, diarrhoea and respiratory diseases were common. Surprisingly, immunisation coverage was good. As immunisations are the only long-lasting protection which mothers could secure for their children during occasional trips to health centres in Sandinista-controlled territory, they carefully sought them out.

The teams trained *brigadistas* to staff four abandoned health posts and establish 20 new ones. These volunteers will form the core of a rural health service. Private organisations will also be involved in these efforts. The most important is probably CEPAD — the major Protestant social service organisation in the country — which runs dozens of clinics as well as other programmes to feed and house displaced people.[33]

Volunteers treat the local population as well as patients who have brought medical records (complete with *Contra* insignias and flags) back with them from Honduras.[34] They hope to continue building this rural health network as the war winds down. According to Dr. Gavidia, "We have to create the peace now."

Primary care vs. hospital care

The *Contra* war has greatly increased the need for highly skilled surgical care and rehabilitation, which can be provided only through expanded and improved hospital facilities. Until 1983, Nicaragua's health budget increased the share for primary health care and reduced the proportion for hospital care. Since 1983, however, the proportion allocated to hospital care has increased in order to cope with the influx of war-related injuries requiring hospital surgery, and to reduce the deterioration of hospital services.

It appears that the war led to a retreat from community-based, primary health services with an emphasis on prevention. Greater reliance on the skills of hospital-based surgeons and other medical specialists became the norm. Yet where doctors cannot provide modern curative care, as in the war zones and other remote areas, a renewed reliance on volunteers and preventive activities has occurred. With the war, a two-tiered system of care emerged — a rural system run by *brigadistas* at the primary care level and an urban system led by surgeons and other specialists needed for war-related pathologies.

Yet while the curative hospital system was being strengthened in cities, the resources of the entire health system were being stretched to breaking-point. The military and economic war against Nicaragua had, by the mid-1980s, plunged the health system into a deep economic and organisational crisis.

Chapter 7: From Expansion to Crisis Containment: 1983 - 1989

"The truth is that we have made errors. One of these was the big expansion plans we had for the health sector. It was right to bring health services to the whole population, but not to try to do it all immediately, overnight."
(President Daniel Ortega, 1985)[1]

When there was a national shortage of light bulbs in 1985, hospital nurses on their nightly rounds carried a bulb with them from ward to ward. It seemed that everything — supplies, equipment, spare parts for vehicles, fuel, and food for patients — was either in short supply or not working. Articles appeared in local newspapers denouncing the theft of medicines by MINSA officials. Articles also started to appear in the international press about the collapse of the health system.[2] It hardly seemed possible that this was the same country which, in 1982, received recognition from the World Health Organisation for its achievements in primary health care.

WHO's interest in the Nicaraguan health 'model' was fitting acknowledgement of the momentous changes that occurred during the first few years of the Sandinista revolution. Between 1980 and 1983, government health expenditure in Nicaragua averaged $40 per person annually — triple the level of spending prior to 1979.[3] Hospitals were opened to the entire population, hundreds of health posts were constructed, thousands of health workers were trained and nation-wide prevention programmes were begun. Community organisations set health priorities and carried out programmes.[4] Tens of thousands of volunteers organised health activities. Yet these many initiatives were often anarchic in character.[5] A way was urgently needed to bring them together in a coherent national primary care programme.

PIASS

In April 1983 such a programme was launched as PIASS, 'The Integrated Programme for Activities in the Health Area'. PIASS consisted of 18

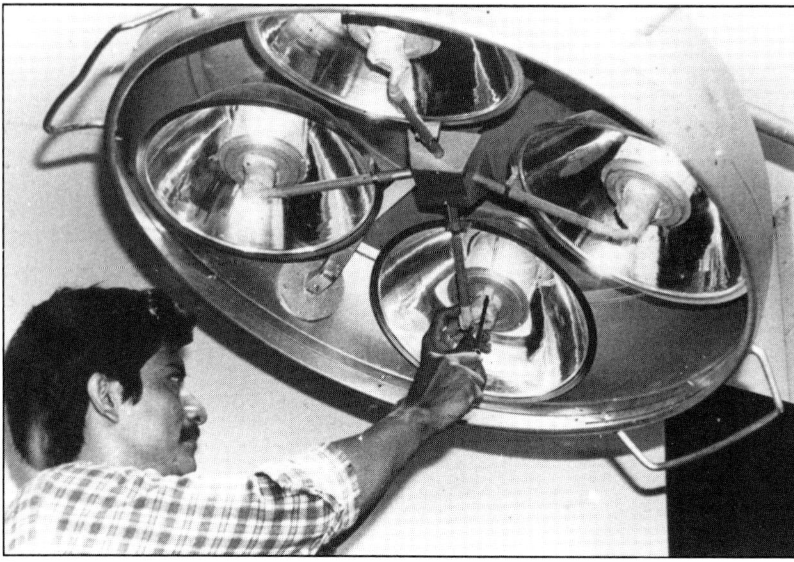

EL NUEVO DIARIO

Because of a shortage of high intensity surgical light bulbs, an ordinary light bulb is adapted for use instead.

specific disease control programmes with an emphasis on prevention. This was an attempt to take clinic-based services into the community.[6] MINSA hoped that the new system would foster community participation in, and demand for, health services. PIASS was also expected to establish links with literacy programmes, combat childhood diseases, improve housing and nutrition, and generally raise the quality of people's lives.[7]

PIASS had four distinctive features. First, it aimed to ensure that doctors would be available at health posts so that professional health services could extend from the clinic to neighbourhoods and villages. Second, PIASS programmes would be carried out by interdisciplinary teams of health workers. The primary health programme was to involve a total of 18 disease or risk-group-specific activities. Third, health volunteers (including trained birth attendants) were to be members of the team at health centre or post level. Finally, the programme was to emphasise the importance of living conditions (housing, water, sanitation, hygiene) as determinants of health. PIASS (along with DECOPS, see Chapter 4) was expected to help communities examine the causes of disease and ill health in the social and political context of their communities in order to motivate local efforts for change.

The programme began in Esteli, where the revolution had strong support and community organisations were very active. It was further tested in five of the 17 health areas of Managua in early 1983. Later that year, despite warnings from some health leaders to avoid hasty

Fig. 7.1

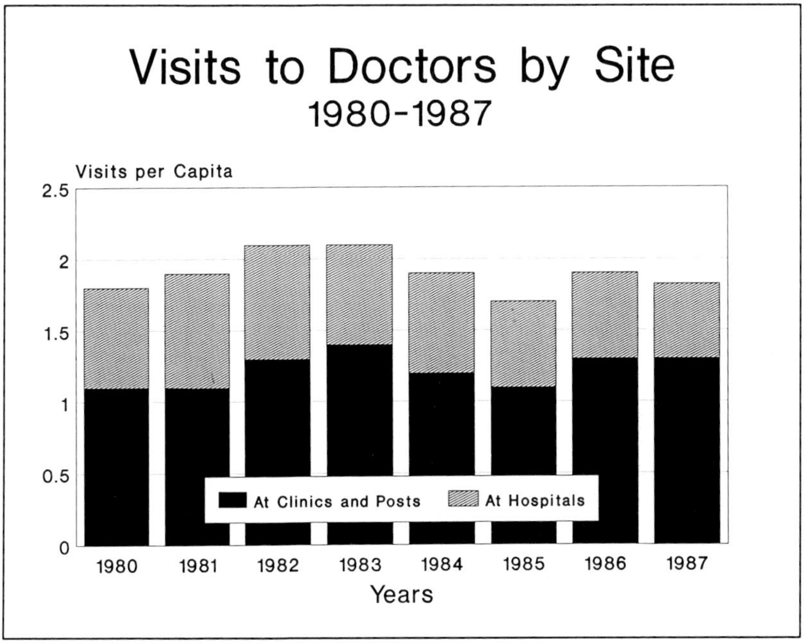

Per capita medical visits declined between 1982 and 1985. They rose again in 1986 when new efforts in primary care were made. Throughout the decade the percentage of all visits occurring at hospitals declined.

implementation, it was proclaimed the nationwide programme for primary care.

Health leaders hoped that the enthusiasm with which PIASS had been taken up in the pilot areas would be replicated nationally. The economy was growing, the health sector was still relatively well-endowed with funds, and the *Contra* war was only just starting to drain the country's limited resources. Health professionals and community leaders were also euphoric about the recent participation of tens of thousands of volunteers in mass campaigns against malaria, dengue, polio and measles (see Chapter 5). It seemed that anything could be done.

It soon became evident, however, that PIASS made impossible demands on the country's limited resources. The scheme did capture the imagination of many health professionals, community leaders and volunteers. They believed that the improved health which PIASS would engender would reduce demands on the curative care system. Instead, it led to new demands and expectations for doctors and medicines which the health system could not meet. In 1983, the year when PIASS was launched nationally, the average number of visits to a doctor per person

Fig. 7.2

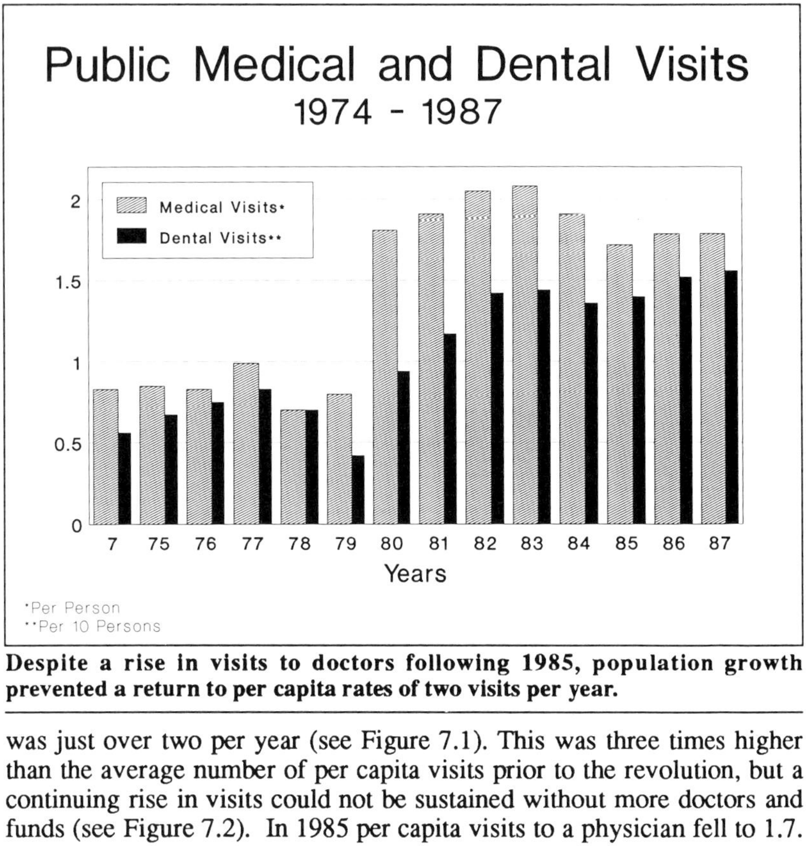

Despite a rise in visits to doctors following 1985, population growth prevented a return to per capita rates of two visits per year.

was just over two per year (see Figure 7.1). This was three times higher than the average number of per capita visits prior to the revolution, but a continuing rise in visits could not be sustained without more doctors and funds (see Figure 7.2). In 1985 per capita visits to a physician fell to 1.7. The decline in medical visits was partly a result of the closing or destruction of facilities by *Contras*.

With the *Contra* war draining government resources and the economy beginning to decline, PIASS faltered. But the haste with which PIASS was introduced, with insufficient resources or planning, also reduced its chances of success. With inadequate training and little information about the new system, many health workers did not even fully understand how PIASS was supposed to work.

The Health Plan for 1987 admitted,[8] "[PIASS] was planned on the basis of international norms without consideration of the national reality. It was planned to implement an endless number of programmes, each of high priority, in thc health areas, without careful consideration of the fact that, at the present time, only nursing personnel are available at this level [the health post]."

The critical weakness of PIASS was that it assumed that there would

Fig. 7.3

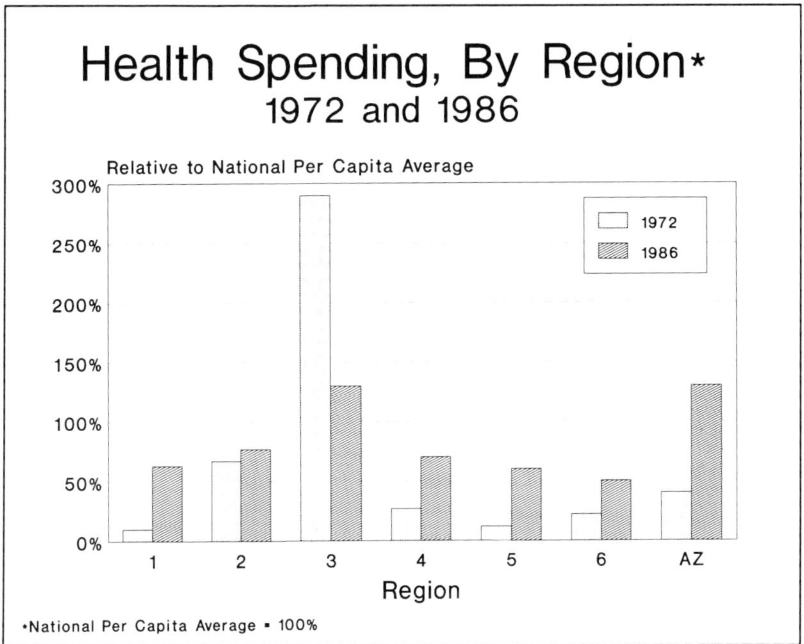

In 1972 health funding was highly concentrated in the capital city of Managua. By 1986, per capita spending was far more equitable.

be enough revolutionary doctors and funds to staff a high quality system of primary care. As will be shown later, neither the doctors (see Chapter 10) nor the funds (see Chapter 12) materialised. Primary health care continued, but services were less accessible, less community-oriented, and less preventive than was envisioned in the programme. The PIASS name fell into disuse and was not heard of after 1985.

Quality of care

During the early 1980s Nicaragua's political leaders encouraged the public to expect free health care as one of the fruits of the revolution. It was therefore hardly surprising that people demanded more and better health services, especially hospital care. By 1983 the country's health leaders were forced to admit that the quality of the health services was often poor and getting worse.

From 1979 to 1983, MINSA allocated increasing resources to primary care. This resulted in a much fairer distribution of health resources between Managua and outlying regions (see Figure 7.3). But the inevitable consequence was that hospitals, which had already suffered from neglect during the Somoza regime, declined more rapidly. Staff salaries were frozen and little incentive for educational advancement existed. Chronic supply shortages became more severe, and long neglect of maintenance led to the deterioration of physical plant.

Many hospitals had running water only part of the day, electricity failed during surgery, and back-up lights broke down. On three separate occasions in a single year, a surgeon in Esteli hospital was left in the dark with a patient's abdomen wide open during a gastro-intestinal operation. Whenever the electricity failed or respirators in an intensive care unit broke down, a nurse had to maintain the oxygenation of the patient by hand, sometimes for as long as 24 hours.[9]

Dr. Antonio Dajer helped perform an operation for retained gall stones and an infected gall bladder under these conditions. "Without cautery, intra-operative X-rays, or even the right-sized drain, we plunged in. I could barely tell the gall bladder from the liver or small intestines, the scar tissue was so thick. The operation lasted five hours. Half-way through the power went out. An emergency generator kept a light on, but there was no air. Beneath heavy surgical gowns, sweat soaked my underwear. My glasses threatened to slide off my nose. The scrub nurse fainted, but the patient's vital signs remained steady."

Some of the older hospitals had a mediaeval atmosphere about them. The wards were long, dark chambers, in which two patients often had to share a single bed. Psychiatric patients wandered freely across dirt courtyards, dogs and children scavenged in garbage heaps, while laundry women scrubbed blood-stained hospital sheets over open-air concrete sinks.

Three of the worst hospitals were closed when five new ones came into service between 1981 and 1984. Financial constraints made it necessary to shelve plans for other new hospitals and clinics. Instead, emergency repairs were carried out to keep old facilities in use. Hospital salaries were also increased in 1983 to attract larger numbers of qualified doctors and nurses. Personnel and resources were shifted from primary care to hospitals in the hope that the quality of hospital care would improve within two or three years. The war intervened, however, depriving the health system of human and material resources, and giving a further twist to the downward spiral in the quality of hospital care.

With rapid population growth and no new hospitals being built, the bed-to-population ratio fell behind the rate of population growth (see Figure 7.4). The Pan American Health Organisation goal of 4.5 beds per 1,000 population slipped farther and farther out of reach. Lack of funds to buy or repair equipment meant that even investments in the new hospitals sometimes did not translate into more or improved care. At best, the shift in funding from primary care to hospitals only slowed the deterioration.

To make matters worse, many people continued to use hospitals as primary health centres. They had heard that hospitals once again were

Fig. 7.4

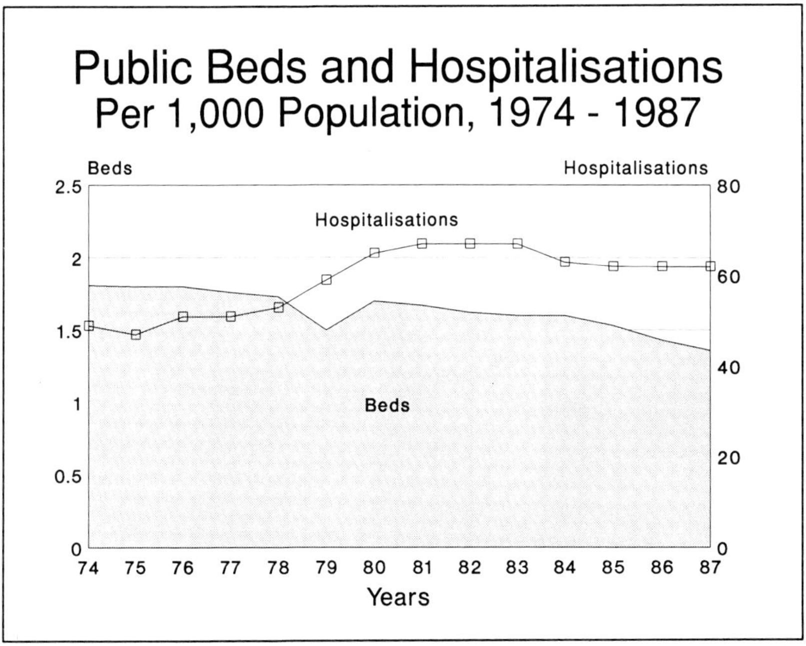

Although the rise in hospital beds has not kept pace with the rise in population, beds are being used more intensively and the rate of hospitalisations has increased.

receiving a greater share of health funds. As a result, the increased funds were used to keep up with increased demand for services. Doctors commonly saw 12 patients per hour in hospital clinics. This gave them little chance to do more than write prescriptions and make a short note in the chart. The funds and time needed to repair the buildings and improve the quality of care at hospitals never materialised. Yet while patients with routine illnesses started queuing up outside hospitals at 3 a.m., urban health centres and posts sometimes were without clients.

Matters came to a head in June 1985, when President Daniel Ortega, along with the Ministers of Health, Finance, and Transport, and other Cabinet members, faced 500 doctors in a lively question-and-answer session in Managua. The doctors voiced their grievances over problems such as salaries, taxes, housing, vehicles, supplies of medical equipment and drugs, and the deplorable state of public hospitals. President Ortega was brutally frank in admitting the failures of the new health system:[10]

"We spread out to build hospitals in every direction...without taking realistic account of our human and financial limitations...The hospitals we built are open, but without the staff to make them work, they are functioning at only 20% or 30% capacity."

To make matters worse, public confidence in MINSA was shaken by the discovery in 1985 that several officials in Managua had stolen quantities of valuable pharmaceuticals to sell them on the black market.[11] Morale was low and solutions to pressing problems in the health system were elusive.

A change in leadership

It was against this background that, in July 1985, Health Minister Lea Guido was replaced by 31-year-old military commander Dora Maria Tellez. Before joining the FSLN in 1974 Tellez had been a second-year medical student. An inspirational leader and efficient organiser, she rose quickly to become a high-ranking political and military figure. She seemed well-suited to the challenges of restoring staff morale and overhauling the system of health administration. Many doctors, however, feared that she would impose military-style solutions on MINSA. The opposition newspaper, *La Prensa*, had more trivial concerns, twice pointing out in its first article on the new Minister that she did not wear make-up during the interview.[12]

Tellez surprised and impressed her critics with a professional approach and clear sense of priorities. She tightened national administration through her personal involvement in many technical matters. Accountability improved dramatically. At the same time, many decision-making powers and personnel were transferred to the regions.[13] Most regional health directors established contact with the Minister's office each day.

Tellez's tenure at MINSA began with a review of the previous six years' work. When the Sandinistas came to power in 1979, they promised free, universal access to doctors and hospitals. In the rosy afterglow of the revolutionary insurrection, this promise did not seem unrealistic. It was, after all, what people expected of a revolutionary government. But it was a promise based on three crucial assumptions: first, that the economy would recover rapidly; second, that large-scale international aid would be available; and third, that most doctors would remain in the country.

In practice, none of these assumptions proved true. The economy, after an initial recovery, declined rapidly after 1983. Large-scale international aid for health and development was limited after 1980[14] (see Chapter 12). Some 300 doctors, including many of the most highly qualified specialists, left the country by 1982, leaving gaps in specialty care. A fundamental reappraisal of the sort of health system that Nicaragua could realistically afford was needed.

In the first few years of the revolution, MINSA's policy was to provide the most advanced care available to the poor majority. Some argued for a cheaper and more limited approach to primary care based on low-cost technological inputs, community participation and an inter-sectorial approach to health. Indeed, the revolution's most successful health programmes — malaria control, polio and measles immunisation, and promotion of oral rehydration therapy — had used such low-cost health technologies and involved tens of thousands of non-professional health workers.

But many leaders, including those in MINSA, were suspicious of this approach. Such suspicions were reflected in the attitude toward the community health manual *Where There Is No Doctor*, the most widely used clinical reference text for auxiliary health workers in the developing world:[15] "We were told," recalled one young doctor, "to go ahead and use it if we wanted to, but officially speaking it was neither needed nor wanted. Our health leaders thought that such a simple, basic book was shameful in a top-notch public health system like ours."

By the mid-1980s, however, such attitudes had changed. Even without the drain on human and material resources caused by the *Contra* war and the economic crisis, Nicaragua simply could not afford a health system based on highly trained doctors and sophisticated hospitals.

This realisation led to a revised health strategy, more appropriate for a developing country with a rapidly growing population but dwindling resources. The Health Plan for 1987 stressed the importance of "the wider search for, and application of, low-cost, simple, alternative technologies".[16]

In a speech to the National Student Organisation in 1987, President Daniel Ortega went further: "We aren't thinking about medical care for a developed country, but about minimal care for our population. But we don't have even the resources to pay for the medicines, maintain the hospitals, and keep all the operating theatres and recovery rooms working. We have to create a survival economy in health."

By 1988, MINSA openly embraced the concept of low-cost health technology. The plan for the 'Campaign to Defend Children's Lives', for example, stresses the need "to promote cost-appropriate water projects, especially in rural areas". Minister Tellez, addressing the need for latrines, said:

"Any kind of latrine is better than defaecating in the open air. If we don't have the resources to make latrines with good seats, even just a simple hole in the ground will suffice. We have to be ready to meet our needs with whatever minimal resources are available, and not wait for better conditions."

A 'survival economy' approach to health did not mean a return to the choice between third-rate medicine or no medicine at all.[17] Instead, it attempted to adapt effective, inexpensive modern medical technologies to the country's most common and urgent problems. One example is the strategy for attacking cervical cancer, the most common cause of cancer deaths among adult women.

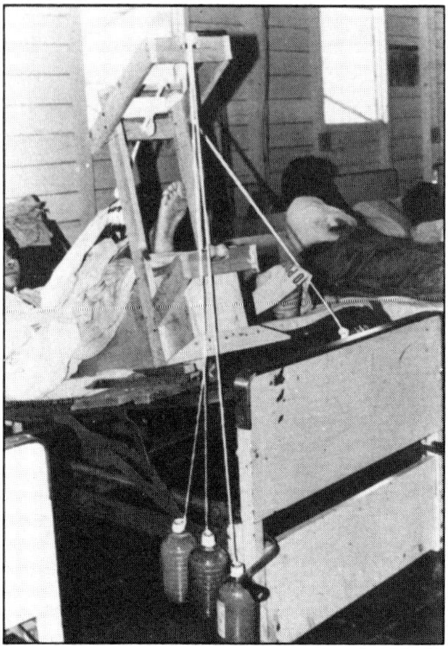

EL NUEVO DIARIO

Low-cost health technology in action — a makeshift traction apparatus for a fracture patient at the hospital in Apanas, Region 6.

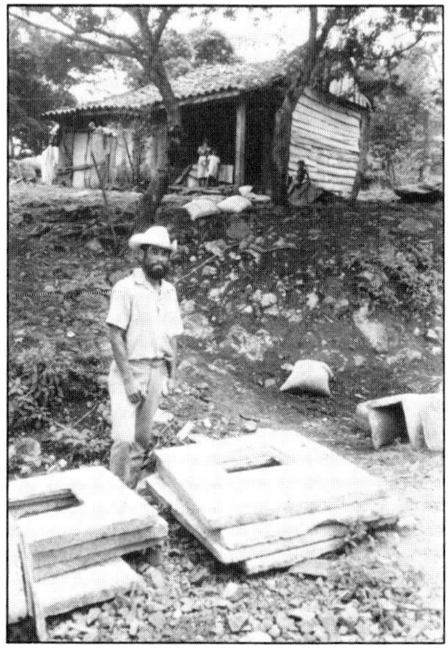

RICHARD GARFIELD

A health *brigadista* with latrines to be installed in his village, 1988. The Government has provided the materials and the people of the village will build the latrines.

Nicaraguan cancer specialists have long wanted to build a specialty hospital to diagnose and treat a wide variety of cancers. Such a hospital would be enormously costly, but would bring only limited benefits since a long-term cure is still unavailable for most cancers. Cervical cancer, however, can often be cured if discovered early. It accounts for about 40% of the cancers diagnosed among Nicaraguan women and occurs most frequently among women in their reproductive years.

Rather than build a cancer hospital, MINSA is building a pavilion attached to one of the hospitals in Managua to treat cervical cancer patients.[18] The specialised staff needed to read pathology smears are now being trained, and adequate equipment for a large-scale national screening programme is being procured. This is a far more modest project than the originally planned cancer hospital. It is, nonetheless, likely to bring many benefits, much sooner, and at greatly reduced cost.

Using hospitals

In 1986, medical students carried out a review of seven national referral hospitals in Managua. Their findings reveal the incredible difficulties under which care was provided [see box]:

Most patients treated at hospital emergency and outpatient departments

Conditions in four Managua hospitals, 1986

Antonio Lenin Fonseca Hospital, the surgical referral institution:
"The hospital was built for 150 beds, but currently has double that number. Many patients must sleep in the hallways. Air conditioning often does not work in the surgical suites, necessitating open windows."

Manolo Morales Peralta Hospital, the internal medicine referral institution:
"Desperately needed items included elastic bandages and gauze, tape, plaster, and EKG paper. Because the laundry equipment was in poor repair, sheets had to be dried outside, spread out on the grass. During the rainy season, there are few dry sheets."

Berta Calderon Hospital, the referral obstetric institution:
"Intensified use of maternity services meant that scrub uniforms were washed and reused four times a day."

Fernando Velez Pais Hospital, the referral maternal-child institution:
"Of 135 routine items which should be available at all times, only 15 were currently available. Of 480 pharmaceutical products expected at all times, 164 were never available."

could be treated better at health centres or posts. A study in Manolo Morales Hospital, for example, found that 70% of patients treated in the emergency department had no medical need to bypass their local health centre. Primary care personnel, under less pressure from long queues of patients, could actually provide more attention and better care than overworked hospital staff.

Nicaragua's pluralistic system of overlapping care from the primary care system, private doctors and public hospitals has encouraged patients to go 'hospital shopping' — taking treatment at several institutions at the same time for the same illness. This practice was given a new dimension by war-related shortages of staff, equipment, drugs and supplies.

Even the most basic of laboratory tests may be unavailable from a regional hospital, but obtainable (at a stiff price) from the private sector. Many urban residents have become sophisticated 'hospital shoppers', using various types of care in combination. They may go to a private laboratory to have a blood test done, then take the results to the outpatient department of a government hospital. If the illness requires only supportive care, they may go to a private clinic or hospital. If surgery is required, they will probably go to a public hospital.

Fig. 7.5

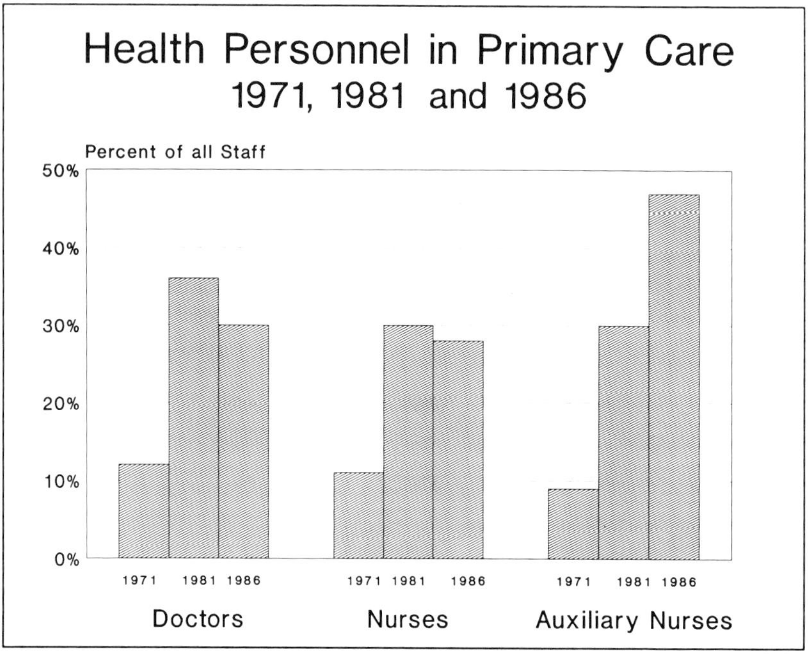

Most of the rise in numbers of nurses and doctors working in primary care following the revolution was maintained at least until 1986. By 1986 auxiliary nurses were the most numerous type of health worker in primary care.

Rural health services

Almost all communities of more than 5,000 residents in Nicaragua now have a health centre or health post. Although the construction of new health facilities has been severely curtailed since 1984, many communities have managed to build and equip their own facilities, often assisted by non-governmental agencies in Europe and North America.

Equipment, however, is also in short supply in rural areas. A typical day at a rural health post begins with resterilising equipment used during the previous day. Needles are reused until they are dull enough to be heard breaking the skin. If gloves are worn out and likely to break during a procedure, two pairs are worn.

Despite such limitations, rural health care remains a clear example of the commitment and effectiveness of government-led services. The proportion of personnel dedicated to primary care remained high throughout the 1980s (see Figure 7.5). The rural health centre in El Cua is typical of those in rural areas with a dispersed population. Established in what was one of Somoza's jails, the centre was set up with Italian

Fig. 7.6

Health Resources
Public, Private and Military, 1987

	Public	Private	Military
Beds	4786	200	480
Hospitals	31	7	3
Health Centres	100	150**	*
Health Posts	390	--	*
Pharmacies	61	275	*

*Not Available **Including Doctor's Offices

Source: MINSA, *Plan de salud 1988-1990*, Managua: MINSA, 1988.

assistance in 1981 and now provides more than 50,000 consultations each year to the 35,000 people living in the area. It has a staff of three doctors, two graduate nurses and ten auxiliaries. Five health posts refer patients to this centre. Two of these posts have been destroyed, and the centre itself was attacked in 1983. Despite the isolation of the population and the war-related destruction suffered by the health system, primary care services are stable and remain widely available. The nearest advanced health facility is 80 kilometres away in Jinotega.

What makes up the 'unified national health system'?

During the 1980s, health services have evolved into a system with several overlapping components (see Figure 7.6). The Ministry of Health directly provides an estimated 70% of all health services through its 31 hospitals, three polyclinics, 105 health centres, and 500 health posts.[19]

An East German and a Soviet-run hospital, under Ministry of Health direction, provide some of the more specialised care available within the country. Separate health facilities run by the Army and the Ministry of the Interior provide health services for the armed forces and the police respectively. It is generally thought that these facilities provide the best surgical care in the country.

The private sector is also an important provider of care, particularly ambulatory care. It consists of doctors' surgeries and clinics, private hospitals, pharmacies, and many small shops selling medicines. Doctors have even started to open 'mini-hospitals' in their private clinics. These

Fig. 7.7

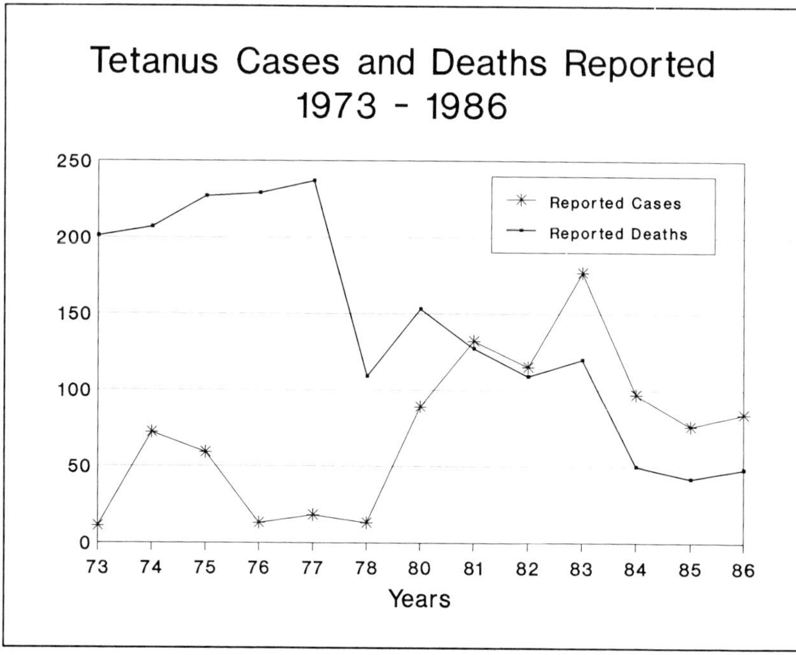

Under-reporting of diseases in the 1970s was so bad that there were more deaths from tetanus reported than cases. Only after a new vital statistics system was developed following the revolution, were more cases than deaths reported.

are popular with middle or upper-class people. Perhaps as many as 90% of physicians maintain some type of private practice. A number of factories and farms employ doctors on a part-time basis. Even some government ministries offer on-site medical services provided by a private physician as a perk for their employees. Dozens of church-run clinics and a Baptist hospital are also major sources of care.

The 1988 Health Plan reflected on this situation:[20]

"At this moment, there is no health system in the strict sense. What exists is a combination of uncoordinated subsystems with diverse objectives, priorities, and technologies."

MINSA provides the administrative coordination to maintain these subsystems. Facilities in most health areas, whether public or private, depend on the government for transportation, coordination, supply, referral, and personnel. More importantly, MINSA provides political and technological leadership to shape and modify the subsystems, set priorities, and influence action on health-related issues in other sectors of society.

Fig. 7.8

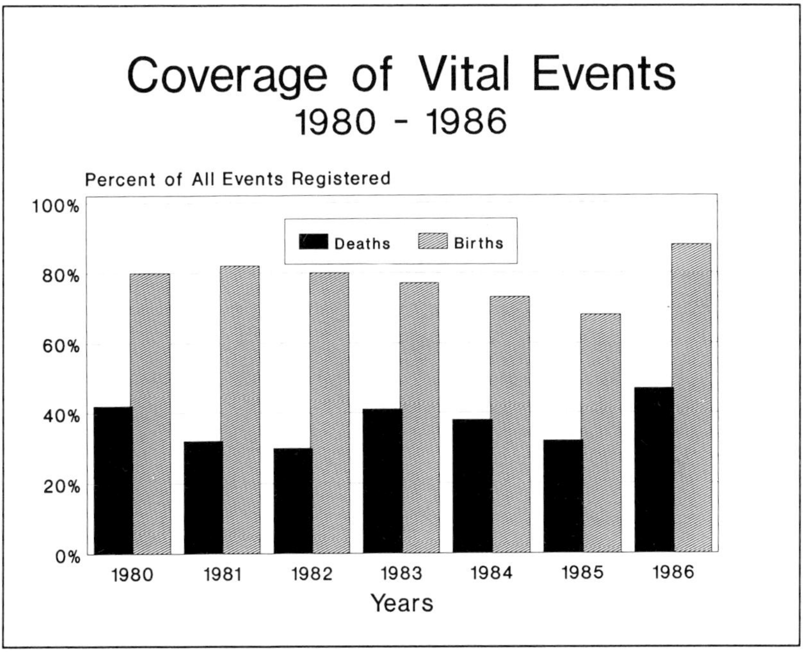

Births and deaths recorded are compared to the estimated number of births and deaths in the country. Reporting on births is much more complete than reporting on deaths. The quality of reporting for both vital events declined from 1983 to 1985, and began to improve again in 1986.

Health information

"When you fill out this form you make it possible for Nicaragua to know her children so that she can care for them." (MINSA Vital Statistics Training Manual)

Many vital statistics (births, deaths, outbreaks of epidemics) go unregistered, providing policy makers and planners with inadequate information.[21] Until 1983, for example, more tetanus deaths than total tetanus cases were reported (see Figure 7.7). Although MINSA trains and employs registrants in all regions, the war has limited their effectiveness. Despite the inauguration of a vital statistics system of national scope in 1983, the percentage of the estimated total births that are actually recorded fell from 80% in 1980 to 68% in 1985 (see Figure 7.8). Similarly, the percentage of all deaths recorded by the vital statistics system fell from 42% in 1980 to 32% in 1985. The situation has improved since 1986, and information on the specific causes of death among the registered deaths has improved steadily year by year. But there are often not enough paper or pencils available for staff to record

Fig. 7.9

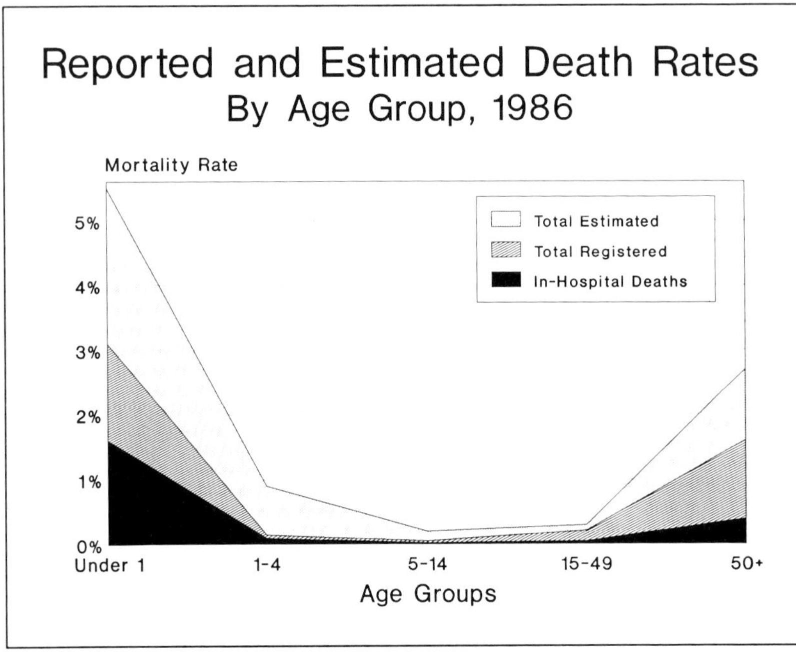

Deaths in hospitals are compared to total deaths reported in the country and the number estimated to have occurred. Most deaths occur among those under one year of age or over fifty. In each of these groups, a high proportion of all deaths occur outside hospitals and are not reported.

vital events. Due to a paper shortage, annual summaries of health service data have not been published since 1983.

Most deaths occur among children under the age of five or adults over the age of 50. It is also among these groups that mortality reports are poorest. About half of all registered deaths occur in hospitals (see Figure 7.9).

Diarrhoea and respiratory infections remain the first and second most common causes of death among children under five years of age.[22] Violence is the most common cause of death among the otherwise low-mortality groups aged 5 to 49 years. Circulatory diseases are the most common cause of death reported for those aged 50 and older (see Figure 7.10). While the projected death rate for each of these disease groups is higher in Nicaragua than the US, the difference in rates is particularly striking for diarrhoea, respiratory diseases, perinatal conditions, nutritional conditions, and unknown causes (see Figure 7.11).

In 1983, the Epidemiology Office began to collect immediate reports of a group of diseases with epidemic potential.[23] Each region now reports

Fig. 7.10

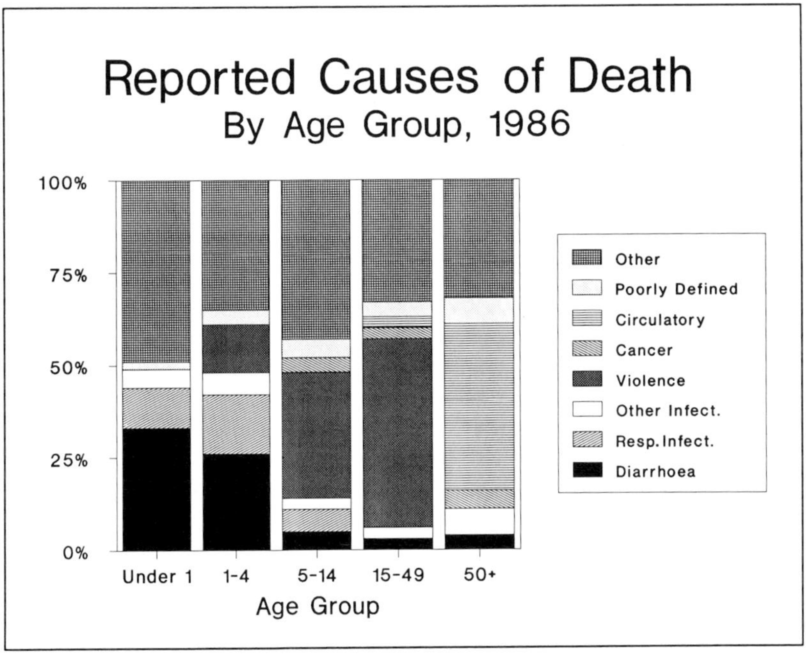

A cause of death is recorded for most reported deaths. While diarrhoea is a major cause of death among young children and circulatory diseases are a major cause of death among those over fifty, serious under-reporting of deaths in these age groups limits the utility of these data.

Source: DINEI, MINSA

suspected cases of diseases such as measles, malaria, tetanus, and typhoid at least once a week to the national office. While this 'vigilance' system has greatly improved the availability of relevant information, data received from some regional offices are still poor. Health areas started to report to their regional offices only in 1986, but 30% of them still do not provide regular reports because of a lack of telephones.[24]

AIDS

The AIDS epidemic presents a new threat to Nicaragua's over-stretched health services. By February 1989 a total of 32 people had tested positive for the HIV antibody; 21 of these were former intravenous-drug users from Europe. About 13,000 blood donors and 12,000 people in high-risk groups have so far been tested for the HIV virus using the ELISA method. Three of the 11 Nicaraguans with positive blood tests have since died of AIDS.

Two of those with positive blood tests were haemophiliacs who

Fig. 7.11

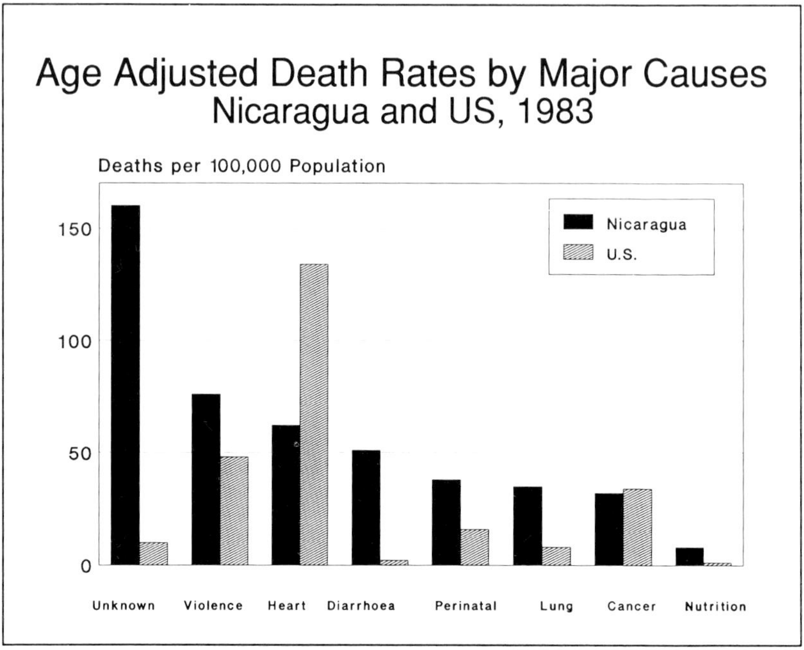

Death rates for diarrhoea, perinatal causes, malnutrition and violence are much higher in Nicaragua than the US. The 'diseases of development' - heart disease and cancer - are higher in the US.

Source: PAHO, Health Conditions in the Americas 1980-84, PAHO: Washington, 1986.

contracted the virus from infected blood products; all other Nicaraguans who tested positive had engaged in high-risk sexual practices. Although there have only been a small number of cases to date, there are adequate grounds for concern. Opportunities for sexual transmission among male homosexuals and bisexuals, prostitutes, and those with multiple sex partners abound. Other sexually transmitted diseases have been increasingly common among these groups, particularly in Managua and Bluefields. If HIV circulates among these groups, AIDS will probably spread rapidly.

A few leaders favour the Cuban approach of widespread screening and quarantine of all those who test positive. A conservative leader of a private medical society argued at an AIDS seminar in 1988: "It works for rabies, so why not do it for AIDS? We are medical professionals here, and we can tell who is and who isn't homosexual. If we round them all up, that will be the end to this problem."

There is, however, far more widespread support for an approach which focuses on educating and organising those at greatest risk. MINSA has begun a campaign to persuade men and couples to use condoms. Starting in March 1989, all motels routinely provide condoms to clients.

The approach to AIDS is surprisingly open. A 'Collective of Popular Educators for the Prevention of AIDS' was formed in 1987. With the assistance of funds and expertise from groups dealing with AIDS in the US, they have trained a network of 25 homosexual and prostitute volunteers in promoting safe sex. Members of this collective have been recruited to the group which sets MINSA policy on AIDS. Workshops on blood testing and safe sex have been held in schools, among prostitutes, and in parks and bars frequented by male homosexuals. Television programmes, health education pamphlets and full-page advertisements in the newspapers openly discuss the means and prevention of transmission.

Decentralisation

MINSA began to reduce administrative centralisation in 1982.[25] Each regional director was freed to determine how to optimise the use of available supplies, personnel and funds. The setting of norms and targets, evaluation and data collection remained national responsibilities, but decisions about how to meet the norms or respond to the evaluation were to be made at the regional level. In practice the change from national to regional decision-making was gradual. Decentralisation received a big push in 1986, when many decision-making powers and personnel were transferred to the regions.

Regionalisation and the use of short (1-2 year) rather than long (5 year) plans have been crucial in reducing the destructive effects of the war and in motivating continued high levels of participation in health activities among volunteer health workers. Without such a radical decentralisation, the flexibility to respond rapidly to local disease outbreaks or military attacks would have been lacking.

Improvements in the medical logistics system have greatly increased the availability of drugs and medical supplies at outlying health centres and posts. This is a major incentive to attend one's local clinic. Most importantly, since 1986 all health centres are staffed by a doctor 24 hours a day in order to improve the local accessibility of care.

An innovative experiment in decentralisation was begun in 1988, when inter-ministerial groups at the regional level began to set health priorities. Regional health authorities were made responsible for coordinating the actions of various government ministries and generating some of the resources for health programmes. In this way, the resources of non-governmental groups, including the church, private industry and international aid organisations, were mobilised more effectively.

The 1988 Health Plan established this pattern of decentralisation as the best solution to the severe lack of ministerial funds. MINSA continues to set norms and evaluate services at the national level, while local areas have more freedom to organise. This includes deciding which types of health personnel to train and utilise, what programmes to stress, and which groups to mobilise. Territorial health systems now have increased flexibility to determine how to relate to private medicine and promote community participation. The system has become most active in outlying regions, where governors and health leaders have a close working relationship.

The main product of the territorial system in Managua is the '*barrio* doctor' programme.[26] In 1987, 20 new graduate physicians were sent to poor neighbourhoods of Managua with great health needs. Doctors were sent only into neighbourhoods where a local resident offered consulting space. They provided ambulatory care in a local home during the mornings and made house-to-house visits with *brigadistas* in the afternoons. Their presence attracted great interest among local residents. Not since PIASS was launched in 1983 had health professionals gone so far outside the clinic door to reach the community. Residents began to compete for the opportunity to host the doctor, local health councils organised the construction of health posts, and *brigadistas* took ongoing responsibility for families targeted for their special health needs. By 1989, 120 physicians were practising in the '*barrio* doctor' programme. Special-care groups, including patients with diabetes, asthma, or hypertension, were set up in some neighbourhoods. Some doctors who were completing their social service considered opening private practices in these high-need areas.

Decentralisation was greatly strengthened when budget cuts forced MINSA to reduce its spending by 10% in 1988 and by 30% in 1989. On both occasions the major cut-back was in administrative staff at the central level. At its peak, MINSA employed 1,000 people at central level. By March 1989 there were only 300.

Conclusions

In contrast to the 'glory days' of 1979 to 1983, the health system has suffered many 'real world' problems between 1984 and 1989. Former Vice-Minister Ivan Tercero views these as two very different stages: "In the first, none of us knew just what to do. All of our efforts were tentative and revisable. By 1984 we had enough training and expertise to establish more stable administration and more comprehensive health programmes. But the resources needed for this work have disappeared. This has forced us to make ever more careful choices."

Falling quality of services, rising public and professional dissatisfaction, and promising programmes gone bureaucratic are among the signs that enthusiasm and good ideas are not enough. The health system did not create the economic crisis of the country, but suffers under it, must cope with it, and tries to protect the population from it. Decentralisation and appropriate technologies for dealing with the country's most common health problems are essential for coping with this crisis.

Another conceivable solution would be the nationalisation of the entire health system and the elimination of private medicine. Such a solution was effective in Cuba,[27] but would probably fail in Nicaragua. First, it would be very expensive. No country has offered Nicaragua the massive funds that such a solution would require. Second, such a top-down approach would probably stifle many of the dynamic processes now at play in the health system. Nicaragua is better-off mobilising the wide variety of public and private resources already in place and making tough choices about health priorities in the new territorial health systems. The next two chapters will explore how these dynamics translate into programmes for the pressing needs of women and children.

Chapter 8: Women's Health

"You can't say now, and maybe you will never be able to say, that the problems of women have been solved. There are enormous problems which have been solved, but there are other great problems which we have not yet begun to address."
(Dora Maria Tellez, Minister of Health, 1 October 1988)

Imagine that you are 30 years old, extremely poor, have four children, and your partner is off in the mountains somewhere. Being 'off in the mountains' could mean several things. He might be fighting with the Army, he might be with the *Contras*, he might be planting beans, or he might just have dropped out of the picture. None of these situations would be unusual: about 60% of Nicaraguan children are brought up by their mothers in single-parent families. You come into a hospital to have your fifth child. You look around at all the people dressed in strange-looking surgical green pyjamas. Which is the doctor, which the nurse, which the cleaning woman? Finally you approach the most sympathetic face and ask the question you've been rehearsing for hours:

"Is it true I can have an operation to stop having kids?" The sympathetic face belongs to a young doctor, who looks at your chart.

"Thirty years old and five children. Yes, you meet the criteria. All you have to do is write a letter to the director and get your husband to sign it."

A particularly painful contraction starts and you wait until it passes before replying: "He's not here."

"What happened to him?" the doctor asks.

"He's in the mountains," you reply.

"Well, you can't get sterilised without his consent. I'm sorry."

The doctor smiles and moves on.

Until recently such scenes were common in Nicaraguan hospitals. Official policy on female sterilisation started to change in 1986, and a male partner's signature is no longer always required. The interpretation of the new policy, however, varies widely from one hospital to another.

A new beginning

Women's health is related to the oppression they have long suffered throughout Latin America. It is manifest in spoken and unspoken rules concerning sexuality and childbearing. When Spain colonised Central America, traditional informal marriage was condemned as immoral, while formal church marriages were available only to the moneyed classes. This left most women without property rights, a stable male partner or full dignity.

The growth of export agriculture and increasing dominance by Hispanic culture further weakened women's economic and social position. A respectable woman did not work outside the home, though her partner might be absent for long periods of time to work on the plantations. Until 1979 any woman seen in public after dark ran the risk of being considered a prostitute. The position of women was worst in rural areas, where most were illiterate, and economically and politically powerless.[1] Domestic violence, rape and abandonment were commonplace in both urban and rural areas. Prostitution was widespread and accepted, even expected, among the poor.

Male chauvinism — *machismo* — finds its clearest expression in the area of sexuality. Women are often not even permitted control of their bodies, as *machismo* demands that men have as many male children as possible. Concern for the health of mothers comes last. Dr. Susan Cookson, who works in a health centre in Jinotega, often sees the results: "Last week I saw a 20-year-old mother of four. She has been taking birth control pills for a year to avoid pregnancy, but she is terrified that her husband will find out. She asked for an intra-uterine device (IUD), but insisted that I must cut the string too short. If she can tell that the IUD is intact, so can her husband. What should I do? She can't handle another pregnancy, but she would be beaten or abandoned if he knew she used contraception."

The revolution promised women a new beginning in health. The Maternal and Child Health programme was the first long-range initiative announced by MINSA in 1979. It included activities related to care during pregnancy and delivery, the detection and treatment of cancer (mainly breast and cervical), fertility control, and sex education. Rapid expansion occurred in medical services to women, including prenatal care, hospital deliveries and gynaecological consultations. At the same time, social and legislative changes were implemented to defend and protect women. These included:

- Direct payment of wages (rather than paying the woman's father or husband).
- The institution of 8 weeks' maternity leave and the right to breastfeed at the work place.
- A law prohibiting discrimination against children born out of wedlock.

• A law on patrimony, specifying financial responsibilities for fathers.
• The establishment of a legal office for women to inform them of their new rights and help them to pursue cases.

New laws such as these are essential to improve the health status of women and children. But laws alone can do little. Major social changes are also needed to prevent oppressive and exploitive treatment of women. Since the mid-1980s, many feel that the pace of reform in this area has slowed.

Working overtime at the baby factory

"After I had my baby, all I wanted to do was sleep", said Esperanza Soriano, who at the age of 20 gave birth at the Berta Calderon Hospital in Managua. "The nurses put me in a bed with my baby by my side and I was out like a light. In minutes I was woken up when another new mother and her baby were put in the bed. After a little while, another mother and baby were brought in. 'What's going on?' I said, 'There's not even enough room for the babies, let alone us mothers!' We ended up leaving the babies in the bed, and we lay on the floor — there was just no room."

Double and triple-bedding is common in maternity wards, and mothers are discharged after 8-12 hours if there are no apparent complications. Berta Calderon Hospital, originally designed to handle 20 births a day, has handled 40 to 70 a day since 1979. Prior to 1979 the average woman gave birth to six children. In rural areas a total of seven children was average; in the cities, five was the norm. Following the revolutionary war a baby boom further raised the birth rate.

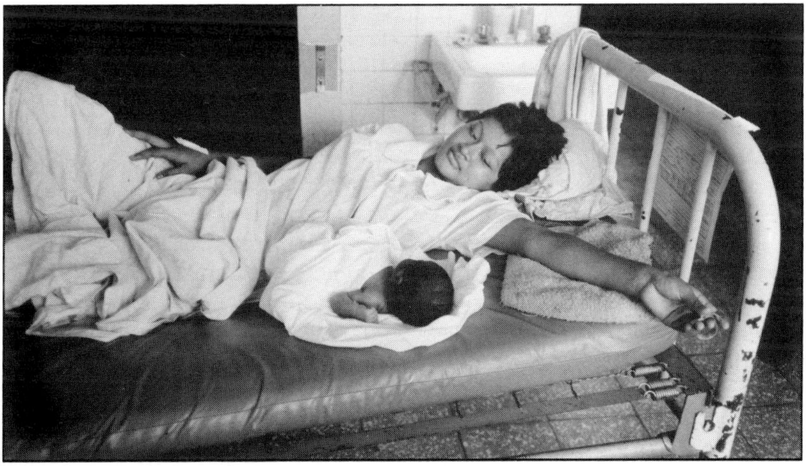

GLEN WILLIAMS

Maternity ward in Oscar Danilo Rosales Hospital, Leon. Many more births now occur in hospitals, but rapid population growth means that the percentage of hospital births has not risen appreciably.

Fig. 8.1

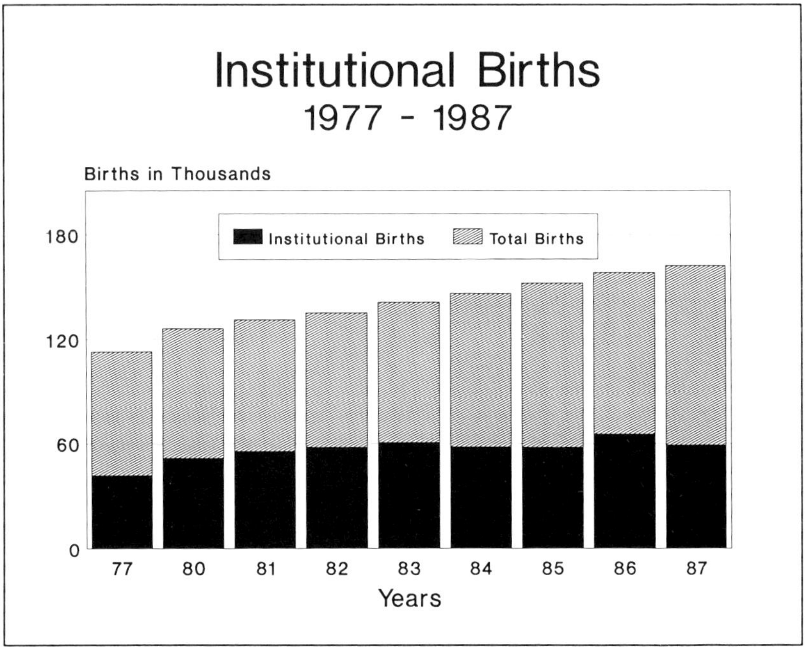

Although the number of births to occur at health institutions rose throughout the 1980s, the total estimated number of births rose much faster.

MINSA made a commitment to have doctors attend all births. In 1980 it set an objective to hospitalise all births within a decade. Before the revolution, 37% of births took place in hospitals. By 1983 the health system handled about 50% more births, but rapid population growth meant that the proportion of births in health facilities rose only modestly, to 43%. By 1985, further population growth and reduced access to health services brought hospitalised births down to 38% of the total — almost the same proportion found prior to the revolution (see Figure 8.1).

Even in Managua, about half of all births still occur at home. In rural areas about 65% of births take place at home. In part this stems from the inherited concentration of maternity services in cities, particularly Managua. There, the two hospitals which attend deliveries are located in the southwest corner of the city, a long distance from most inhabitants. Many women prefer to give birth at home rather than travel a long way under difficult conditions when labour begins.

As the number of births in hospitals increased in the early 1980s, the quality of care dropped. Berta Calderon Hospital became known as the 'Managua Baby Factory'. Hair-raising stories circulated around town of babies being born in the showers, in wheelchairs, and at the admissions desk. The hospital staff, especially doctors, worked under extremely difficult conditions. Stress levels resembled those in a disaster-relief operation. Staff managed to keep their spirits up with the knowledge that conditions in the hospital were still better than those in most homes.

It was not until 1985 that serious reforms in delivery practices began. Health centres in both urban and rural areas were equipped with more beds in order to cater for births. In 1986 health centres began to be staffed by a physician 24 hours a day. Despite these energetic efforts, coverage of deliveries rose only moderately to 41% of all births, while most women delivering at home still did so without trained assistance.

Medical leaders finally admitted that the professional health system was unable to meet the demand for maternity care and accepted that there would be a long-term need to train traditional birth attendants (*parteras empiricas*) to assist women who give birth at home.

The number of antenatal visits has expanded rapidly since 1979, but not all pregnant women receive professional antenatal care.[2] In 1985, a majority of those giving birth in hospitals and half of those giving birth outside hospitals received antenatal care. However, only a third of those giving birth in hospital returned for follow-up care after discharge.[3] It is hoped that better access to postnatal care at health centres will improve this situation. Only a third of all first antenatal visits in 1987 occurred in the first trimester of pregnancy.[4] Among those who receive antenatal care, an average of two visits is made.

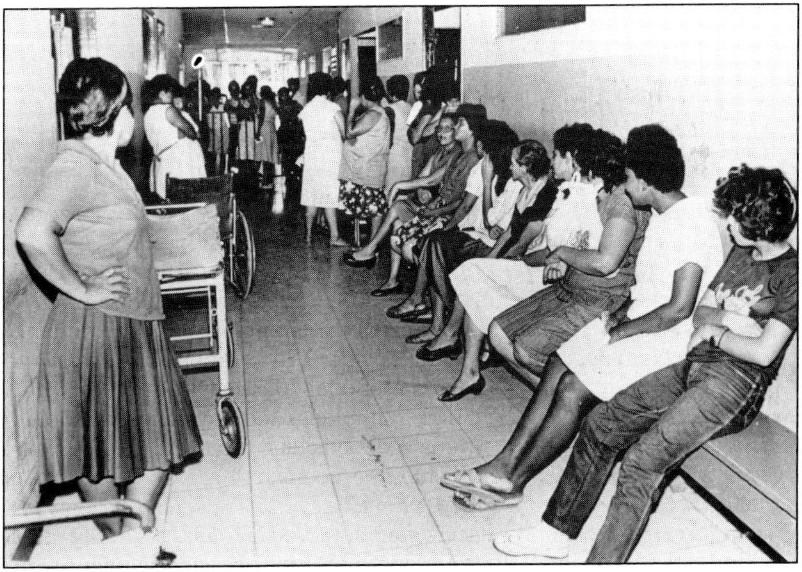

C DONA / EL NUEVO DIARIO

Crowded outpatient department at the Berta Calderon Hospital ('The Managua baby factory'), in 1985.

Contraceptives — now you see them, now you don't

Some military and political leaders still regard contraception as part of a conspiracy by the rich countries to reduce the population of the poor countries of the world. Unfortunately, pre-revolutionary fertility control efforts lend some credence to this jaundiced view. During the 1960s and 1970s about half the international funds for health in Nicaragua were earmarked for fertility control. The pressure to show quick 'results', combined with a lack of concern for people's needs and desires, led to abusive practices such as sterilising women without their consent. A backlash was therefore inevitable. Upon entering Managua in July 1979, a Sandinista commander found a warehouse full of oral contraceptives and ordered them to be burned. Only an emergency petition from the women of the neighbourhood prevented their destruction.

Despite greatly expanded primary health care, most Nicaraguan women still do not have ready access to an effective method of fertility control. Although the number of contraceptive users has grown rapidly during the 1980s, only about one in four women of fertile age uses a method of birth control. Of these, about 80% use oral contraceptives (see Figure 8.2). MINSA estimates that more than half of all women of child-bearing age want contraceptives.[5]

Part of the problem is cultural. In this highly Catholic country, 38% of women interviewed in a national survey in 1985 said that family planning was against the will of God.[6]

Men have long been resistant to using condoms; it is believed that fewer than 5% of men in Latin America use them. *Machismo* prejudices men against the use of condoms because contraceptives reduce the potential number of one's offspring (and therefore, sons). This attitude ignores the pressing health needs of women.

Cervical cancer is the leading cause of cancer deaths among women in Latin America. Condom use would significantly lower the incidence of this disease, yet they are seldom used. The AIDS epidemic and the campaign to persuade people to use condoms to halt the spread of the disease may succeed in changing habits. Dr. Leonel Arguello, Head of MINSA Epidemiology Division, admits, "It's sad to say, but AIDS may be what we need to wake people up. It is the only hope we have for increasing condom use."

Another problem is that oral contraceptives are often unavailable. In January 1986 Dr. Oscar Flores, then Director of Women's Health, went on radio to denounce the warehousing of contraceptive supplies. He alleged that supplies were being withheld by bureaucrats. More than a year later Dr. Marta Norory, Head of Obstetrics at Velez Pais Hospital in Managua, repeated the charge:[7]

"If you go to the central points of distribution the government people will say 'yes, there are contraceptives, here are the lists, here's where they were sent'. I don't know exactly where the system has gone wrong."

Fig. 8.2

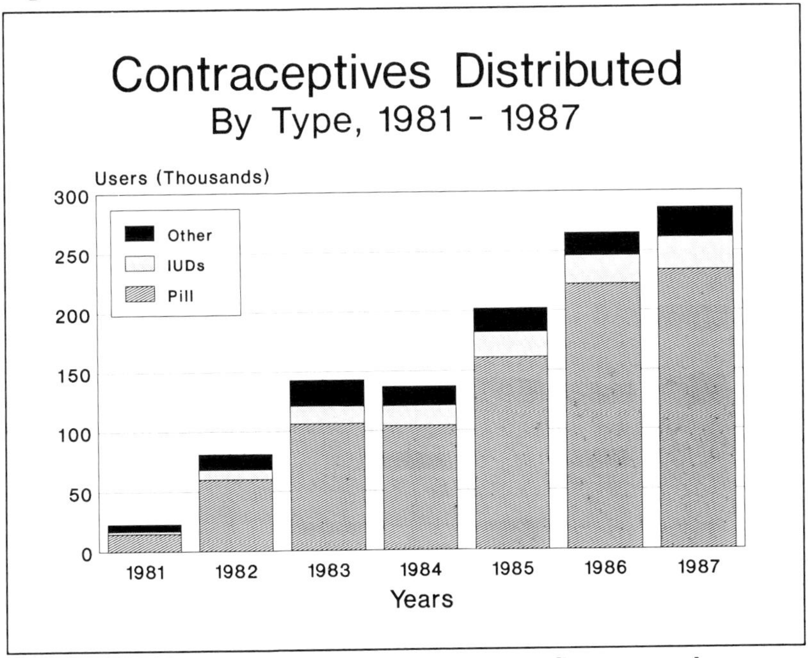

The number of contraceptive users served by the Government has grown rapidly. Most use contraceptive pills.

As a result, many women seeking contraception at health centres are turned away. By the time they return they are looking for ways to end their pregnancies. As abortion is illegal, the government health services can offer little help. In desperation, tens of thousands of women every year resort to other means of terminating unwanted pregnancies.

Abortion

As in most of Latin America, although abortion is illegal it is widely available from private physicians and itinerant abortionists. Said one nurse, "They line up like a queue waiting to use a telephone at a train station." The cost of an illegal abortion is equivalent to four to six months' wages for a manual worker. Minister of Health Tellez says bluntly:

"The truth is that those who can pay for an abortion either have it done abroad or they pay somebody here. The one who has a real problem is the poor woman. She'll fall into the hands of any good-for-nothing."

A common technique of itinerant abortionists is the insertion of a catheter or other rigid object into the uterus to break the amniotic membranes. Women may ask such people to start the abortion in order to arrive at a hospital with an incomplete abortion, knowing they will receive treatment. Those less skilled in using the system, or living far from a hospital, may try to recover alone. In either case, the result is often tragic.

One in every four maternal deaths at the Berta Calderon Hospital in Managua is the result of an incomplete abortion. Complications include sterility, pelvic infections and adhesions, urinary or bowel damage and severe anaemia. And cases treated in hospitals represent only the tip of the iceberg. MINSA treats about 8,000 women after illegal abortions each year. This figure represents only those who reach the health services; it is not known how many more are never seen by a health worker.

The cost of caring for a woman after a poorly provoked abortion is estimated to be 200 times higher than the cost of carrying out a safe procedure. While women suffer as individuals for their inability to control their own bodies, the whole society pays the financial and social costs.

Up to half of all maternal deaths in the developing world may be due to abortions that have gone wrong.[8] These cases contribute to the shocking rates of maternal mortality. About one in every 2,000 births in Nicaragua results in the death of the mother. While infant mortality is about five times higher in Nicaragua than in most developed countries, the death rate among pregnant women is at least ten times higher. This is a measure of how far the revolution still has to go to meet women's health needs.

No reliable estimates of the total number of abortions in Nicaragua exist. Although the number of abortion patients to reach the public hospitals has remained nearly stable,[9] the total number of abortions performed in Nicaragua may have doubled over the last decade.

Dr. Ligia Altamirano led a two-year study on abortion patients at Berta Calderon Hospital.[10] From March 1983 to June 1985, 8,752 women sought care at the hospital for incomplete or septic abortions. About a quarter of these were intentionally provoked. At least ten abortion-related cases arrive daily. Contrary to the prejudiced public image, three-quarters of the women admitted for incomplete abortions were in stable relationships and were raising children.

Dr. Altamirano's study sparked a heated public debate on abortion, sterilisation, family planning, and sex education. This occurred at the time when the National Assembly was drafting a new constitution, and reformers saw this as an opportunity to establish women's legal right to terminate pregnancy. With issues related to abortion in the national press almost every day, a constitutional committee met with women's leaders and other interested parties, including representatives of the Catholic Church. The women's organisation, AMNLAE, was deeply split. AMNLAE leaders caused consternation by declaring that "our women are not ready for the legalisation of abortion", and that "we must concentrate our efforts on sex education and family planning".

Despite impassioned pleas from women in the National Assembly, the constitution was ratified in October 1986 without reference to abortion. AMNLAE has since come out in favour of the decriminalisation of abortion. Until this occurs, most of the abortions seen in the public health system will start as provoked, incomplete procedures. Meanwhile, hospitals are currently permitted to perform abortions only if the life of the mother is seriously threatened.

It is now possible to improve the techniques employed to treat incomplete and septic abortions. In 1987 a training programme began to encourage the use of the manual vacuum aspiration procedure. This technique is used in the only legal abortion clinic in the country. Attached to Berta Calderon Hospital, this clinic charges the equivalent of about two months' wages for the procedure. Dr. Altamirano, for her part, continues to work for women's right to abortion. She doubts, however, whether change will come soon: "The legalisation of abortion?" she asks. "Well, perhaps my daughter will see it."

Traditional birth attendants

According to Minister of the Interior Tomas Borge, traditional birth attendants, or *parteras empiricas*, symbolise Nicaragua as "the land of babies". It has not always been so. In the past, *parteras* were shunned by doctors as superstitious old women. One gynaecologist commented, "Doctors not only were against *parteras*. They found the idea of training obstetric nurse specialists threatening as well." Yet throughout Central America these women provide most of the care to mothers giving birth and to their newborn babies.

In a national survey conducted in 1978, only one in every ten women admitted that she had received care at childbirth by a *partera*.[11] In the more open environment of 1985, the Ministry of Health estimated that 78% of those giving birth outside of hospitals were attended by *parteras*.

When a pregnant woman feels the first labour pains, she calls a *partera*, who goes to the woman's house and stays until a day after delivery. The *partera* takes over the woman's domestic work and supports her through labour. She also anoints the baby, examines the placenta, and buries it outside the house. She may cut the umbilical cord with scissors after tying it off. Others sear the cord with hot metal — a practice that can cause tetanus. Some *parteras* may also advise a mother to restrict her food intake after delivery, thereby contributing to anaemia and lowering the mother's resistance to infection.[12]

In part because of these practices, in part because they were seen as 'profiteers', and in part because they are a threat to the authority of the medical profession, doctors have long ignored or denigrated traditional birth attendants.

In 1976 the Somoza Government, with funding and direction from USAID, ran a programme to train *parteras*. The programme exhibited the weaknesses typical of plans designed in one country and carried out in another. Only 768 *parteras* were identified and trained in two years.[13] Contrary to their tradition, the *parteras* were encouraged to sell medicines. By turning what had functioned as a community service into a business, the programme reduced the attention given to health practices and emphasised the prescribing of medicines and contraceptives. Only one day of the seven-day training programme was devoted to well-baby care and referral of high-risk pregnancies. Most of the course focused on the promotion of contraception. Within two years the programme was ended.

MINSA was initially hostile to the idea of training traditional birth attendants. It was not until 1981, when the Matagalpa regional health authority first began to identify, recruit and retrain them, that the tide began to turn. Although it was proscribed by national policy, the programme caught on and was implemented in Esteli as well. In 1982 national directives were changed to permit the training of *parteras*, thus according them tacit recognition. With the more recent shift to 'appropriate technology' for the 'survival economy' in health, the training programme is being actively promoted.

To many women, *parteras* are not just the most accessible type of maternity care, but also the best. Says obstetrician Dr. Marta Norory,[14] "Someone who is in daily contact with a woman will know her problems, and will be the best person to bring health education to her home and to encourage her to go to her local health centre for more specialised care."

Training of *parteras* now has three main objectives. First, it encourages safe, hygienic delivery practices and discourages potentially harmful ones. Second, it opens a channel of communication with the professional system of health care, facilitating referrals and improved coordination. Third, it involves *parteras* in promoting prenatal care, immunisation, oral rehydration, and well-child home visits. Contraception is included in the training but is not its main focus.

As part of this new programme, *parteras* are encouraged to maintain regular contact with the local health service and to participate in health campaigns. Starting in 1985, training included visits to the obstetric units of hospitals in order to observe institutionalised delivery practices. In some areas, *parteras* are even allowed to attend their clients in the delivery room of a health centre. In Ciudad Sandino, on the outskirts of Managua, *parteras* are part of the local obstetric service.

Many *parteras* initially lacked trust in the government training initiative. They thought they would be punished or ridiculed if they took part. An early organiser of the programme recounted her many difficulties:[15] "When I arrived in Jalapa, MINSA had identified only eight midwives in the entire area of 9,000 urban and 23,000 rural inhabitants. I

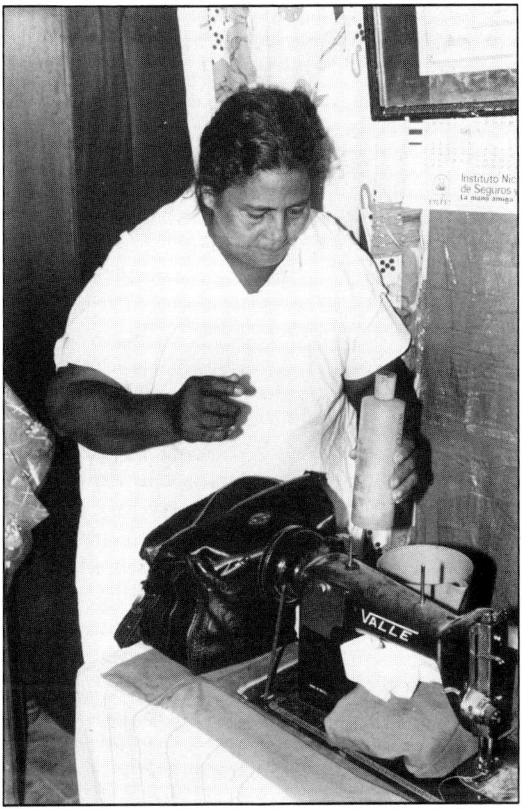

GLEN WILLIAMS

Rita Toruno Mesa, a *partera* from Leon. For many women, *parteras* are not just the most accessible type of maternity care, but the best.

said that if that's all you can find, then there is a poor relationship between the Ministry and the community. I went to the mass organisations and explained the programme...I got the best help from the people, especially the teachers and church workers...and it was beautiful how the mass organisations selected their *parteras* to attend the course...Within ten days the list went from eight to 60 midwives...and the communities organised child care so that they could come to attend the course."

By 1986, close to 6,000 of the estimated 10,000 *parteras* in Nicaragua had been trained. Their training manual states: "In bringing the traditional birth attendant into the heart of the health system...we are making her part of the health team of the area; we are giving her the right, which was formerly usurped, to manifest herself as a person; we are giving her the opportunity to be a participant in the solution of the health problems of her family and of her people."

Most traditional birth attendants are over 50 years old. In 1988 MINSA called for the development of a new generation of *parteras*. In the early days of the programme, auxiliary nurses were responsible for their recruitment and training. Now *parteras* themselves take responsibility for the recruitment and training of others. Slowly, a partnership between midwives and health professionals is emerging.

Sex education

Visits to Nicaragua by feminists from Europe and the United States during the early 1980s typically involved interviews with leaders of the national women's organisation AMNLAE. On many occasions, sex education books such as *Our Bodies, Ourselves*[16] were brought. AMNLAE staff looked at the explicit pictures and studied the frank texts with a mixture of curiosity and self-consciousness. "Thank you for the materials," the foreigners were told, "but we are afraid that they are not quite appropriate for us."

Until recently, it has been almost impossible for women to talk about sex in public. Their understanding of their own bodies has been severely limited. Ignorance of sexual and reproductive matters is still reflected in everyday conversation. Many women talk about men 'having' sex and 'giving' it to women. It is common for Nicaraguan women to say that the man 'gave me a baby'. Most health workers know women who have tried to use birth control pills by inserting them into the vagina. Others who take the pill by mouth believe it should be taken only after sexual intercourse.

In the first six months of 1986, a study of the sexual attitudes and practices of 500 women patients was carried out at the Berta Calderon Hospital in Managua. Most of the women reported never or almost never experiencing orgasm. Many had no idea what the word meant. Most had their first baby before reaching the age of 18. A staggering 95% had never received any form of sex education, and 84% had never used any form of contraception.

Yet attitudes are changing, if only gradually. Minister of the Interior Tomas Borge opened the debate in 1982 during a nationally broadcast speech by unabashedly proclaiming that, among other rights, women had a 'right to sexual pleasure'.[17] Mass media and non-governmental organisations have followed Borge's lead. In 1985, Sistemas Sandinistas, a government-sponsored television station, helped the national Sandinista youth organisation produce a series of 18 video programmes covering topics from puberty to prostitution. It became the second most popular show on TV. The programme on juvenile masturbation was highly praised by Nicaraguan youth groups. The day after the broadcast, however, angry parents flooded a call-in radio show with complaints. As a result, subsequent programmes were broadcast later in the evening, and a non-judgmental video on homosexuality was replaced by one scripted by military doctors who presented homosexuality as a psychological illness.

Non-governmental social service agencies also play an important role in sex education. One such organisation, the Centre for Information and Advisory Services (CISAS), provides a wide range of information on women's health to small groups at rural health posts, factories, churches and schools. With the help of puppets, games, slides, and simple drawings, CISAS teaches women to examine their breasts for tumours, demonstrates the insertion of a diaphragm, and shows how a pap smear is done. Another private social welfare organisation, the Nicaraguan Demographic Association (ADN), provides sex education in schools. The ADN also has a clinic which provides family planning services to the public.

By 1985 the word 'sexuality' had crept into polite conversation. Not everyone, of course, is ready to discuss such issues openly. The Catholic Church still believes that sex education should take place only in the home. By no means all the Church's followers, however, feel confident about teaching their children about sex. "How can I teach my kids about sex?" exclaimed a father of three and a fervent Catholic. "They used to slap our hands when we were kids if they thought we were even thinking about it."

Conflicting attitudes over womens' roles in society also leaves the best approach to sex education less than clear. Said obstetrician Dr. Marta Norory:[18]

"In my opinion we can't have a sexual education campaign like the literacy campaign; you can teach people to read in a few months, but you can't change a whole culture. We need to reach many different layers of society at the same time. How are we to educate school children if their teachers are ignorant?"

A solution will require changed attitudes and better information among the teachers. The Government now plans to make sex education part of the secondary school curriculum. This will be useful, however, only if the health system also responds adequately to widespread demand for methods of controlling fertility.

Women in society

Women's health issues are also those of society as a whole, for the health of future generations of Nicaraguans depends on the health and well-being of today's mothers. As both 'consumers' and 'producers' of health services, women have undoubtedly benefited from Nicaragua's revolution. Yet many women continue to suffer from *machismo*, ignorance and lack of control of their own bodies, domestic violence, and dependence on dangerous and illegal abortions.

To change these conditions will require continued legal and social reform and new attitudes among both women and men. Recognition of the need for such changes — and the commitment to carry them out — has grown slowly since the early 1980s. More radical changes are still beyond the horizon. According to Health Minister Tellez, "Women have to define their own needs, their own sexuality. But these are not the problems of women alone. They are questions for the whole of society."

Chapter 9: Child survival

"It used to be a crime to be young in Nicaragua. You could be punished by death from the National Guard if you were over five or death by 'natural causes' if you were under five."
(Dr. Oscar Flores, former Director of Women's Health, Maternal-Child Health Division)

In August 1988 MINSA launched a national programme to cut infant mortality by half within three years. For a country at war and in the midst of a severe economic crisis, it was a remarkably ambitious initiative. To sceptics it seemed unrealistic, even foolhardy. Others viewed it as a desperate attempt to create a sense of national unity. Many health workers and community leaders, however, welcomed the initiative as a means of giving the health system a much-needed sense of direction and focus.

The first four years of the Sandinista administration were marked by unprecedented gains in child health. The literacy crusade of 1980 reached tens of thousands of mothers, helping them to understand the causes of health and disease and what they could do to protect their children.[1] More food was also available. Basic goods such as maize, beans, flour, milk powder, cooking oil, eggs and kerosene were available at subsidised prices from a growing network of local shops.[2] Many people gained access to improved water supplies, electricity, roads, and sanitation facilities.[3]

Infant mortality — perhaps the most sensitive indicator of a nation's health — fell rapidly. Prior to 1979 it was somewhere between 90 and 120 per 1,000 live births.[4] The rate rivalled those of Honduras and Bolivia as one of the worst in Latin America. By 1983 infant mortality fell to a rate more typical of middle-income developing countries — about 70 per 1,000. This chapter examines how that decline occurred, why progress slowed in the mid-1980s, and what is being done to restore the momentum.

Diarrhoea

"The parade of small coffins tells me that the rains have come." (Dr. Fernando Silva, Director of 'La Mascota' Children's Hospital, Managua.[5])

Diarrhoea remains the number one killer of young children in the developing world.[6] During the 1970s in Nicaragua it accounted for almost 40% of all hospital deaths among under-five-year-olds.[7] The frustrations of treating children with diarrhoea helped turn some young doctors into revolutionaries. Said one young doctor who finished training in 1978:

"Diarrhoea has to do with water, food, nutrition, and people's education. At the hospital we would treat a malnourished child for diarrhoea and send him home to the same conditions. Soon he would be back in the hospital. It would go on like that until he died. This was obviously not a medical problem but a social one. Doctors were part of the problem, because we taught the people that hospitals and dangerous medicines were the answers to their problems."

During the late 1970s, consultants from USAID helped promote the use of oral rehydration salts (ORS) through trained community volunteers.[8] The volunteers, however, lacked credibility since they were not linked to the formal health system. Nor were they encouraged to educate mothers in the prevention and treatment of diarrhoea within the home. Their attempts to sell ORS packets on a commercial basis were a failure: the average volunteer sold only nine packets of ORS per year — enough for four or five days' treatment for one child.

In hospitals at that time, children admitted for diarrhoeal dehydration were routinely treated with intravenous therapy, which was costly and often unnecessary. Food was withheld as a matter of course, a practice now recognised as harmful.

Two months after the Sandinistas came to power a national programme to combat diarrhoea was launched. The programme encouraged treatment and prevention of diarrhoea through improved hygiene, sanitation, clean water supplies, and the promotion of breastfeeding. The main emphasis, however, was on the use of ORS to prevent or treat dehydration caused by diarrhoea. The programme began by training auxiliary nurses to administer ORS.

The curative emphasis of the programme was reflected in the rapid spread of oral rehydration centres (*unidades de rehidratacion oral*), or UROs, throughout the country. The original objective of 225 UROs was reached before the end of 1980. Many were set up in community centres established for the national literacy crusade. Others, particularly in isolated areas, were started in private homes. Most, however, were set up in health posts and health centres. Little equipment was needed: a few benches and chairs, a cot, a weighing scale, a saucepan (for preparing the ORS solution), a number of small cups and spoons, and a supply of ORS packets. By 1986 over 400 UROs were in operation around the country.

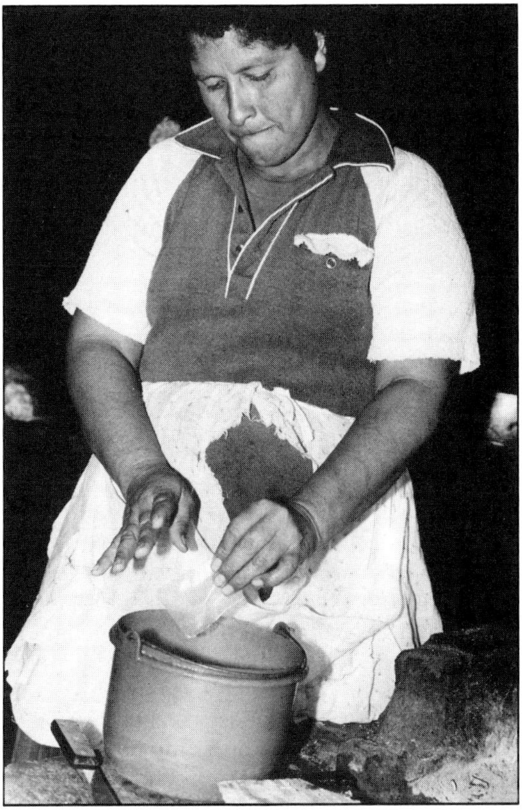

GLEN WILLIAMS

Marixa Arbizu makes up an oral rehydration solution using a packet of oral rehydration salts, in her home in Leon.

Surveys in that year indicated that use of ORS for diarrhoea among children varied from 20% to 50%, depending on the region.

Many communication media were used to educate the public about the dangers and treatment of diarrhoea. In 1980 a half-hour radio programme on diarrhoea was incorporated into the regular broadcasts of the National Literacy Crusade. A 40-second radio announcement repeatedly broadcast the message: "A child with diarrhoea can die. Take yours immediately to the nearest oral rehydration centre." The same message was shown on colourful posters and roadside billboards.

An eight-minute television programme demonstrating ORT and the facilities available at UROs was shown repeatedly at peak viewing times. Newspapers published 200,000 copies of special four-page inserts, in comic strip form, on the causes and treatment of diarrhoea. These were distributed through outpatient waiting rooms, neighbourhood groups, churches, trade unions, adult literacy classes and schools. A flipchart and slide show were also produced for health workers to use in training volunteers and teaching patients.

Meanwhile, paediatric wards in hospitals were undergoing a major transformation. No longer were children admitted for diarrhoeal dehydration routinely put onto an intravenous drip and starvation diet. ORT became the standard therapy, combined with continued feeding. Intravenous therapy was used only for severely dehydrated children unable to take fluids by mouth.

Initial results of this national effort were encouraging. In 1980, 72,000 children were treated at UROs, helping to relieve pressure on the hospitals. At the height of the rainy season in 1980 Dr. Ivan Tercero, then Director of Maternal and Child Health, remarked:

"During the Somoza era the Velez Pais Hospital would be completely filled with children with diarrhoea. This is the first year in which there has been a decrease in severe diarrhoea in this hospital. As a result, we are now able to deal with children who have other problems, such as respiratory infections."

Diarrhoea deaths in hospitals were halved between 1980 and 1982 despite a rise in the number of cases treated. Between 1980 and 1984, diarrhoea fell from the first to the sixth most common cause of infant and child deaths in hospitals. But since only about a quarter of all infant deaths occur in hospitals, this drop had only a limited effect on the country's mortality profile. Diarrhoea remained the most common cause of death among infants nationally.

Many doctors had initially been sceptical about the benefits of ORT. They continued to use anti-diarrhoeal drugs, antibiotics, and intravenous therapy for hospital admissions. But the evidence was clear: the therapy protected against dehydration at low cost and could take pressure off hospitals and clinics.[9]

"Every home a URO"

In 1983 URO nurses were encouraged to give greater priority to teaching mothers how to prepare and administer oral rehydration fluids at home.[10] The health worker was to become more of a teacher than a care-giver. The slogan now was: "Make every home a URO". Most families, however, continued visiting UROs and clinics for supplies of ORS and to seek antibiotic medicines. It was not until 1986 that ORS packets became widely available at a modest price through commercial outlets, thanks to a subsidy from UNICEF. In rural areas where packets are unavailable, health workers promote a home-made solution of sugar and salt.

Between 1979 and 1987 the number of children with diarrhoea seen by the health system more than doubled (see Figure 9.1). In 1987, 264,000 children were treated at UROs — nearly a four-fold increase over 1980. Only 2% received I.V. therapy.[11] The proportion of all children treated for diarrhoea who were treated at UROs increased from 25% in 1980 to 39% in 1986.

Contrary to expectations, however, the demand for doctors' services

Fig. 9.1

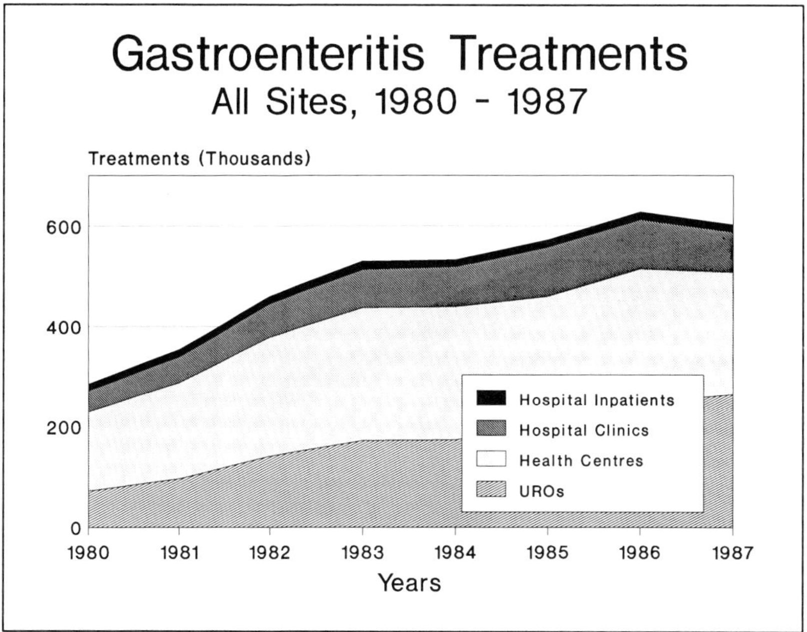

Although the number of children seen at oral rehydration centres (UROs) rose rapidly during the 1980s, even more children with diarrhoea continued to be seen via the primary and secondary health system.

did not decline. Diarrhoea was the main reason for 16% of visits to a doctor in 1986.[12] At least 90% of these children could have been treated more efficiently by auxiliary nurses at an URO. The lure of doctors and hospital-based medicine remains stronger for some people than the convenience of and immediate attention at an URO.

Even more disturbing were the large numbers of children who received inadequate treatment from doctors. A review of 316 diarrhoea deaths in 1985 revealed that 34% had received medical treatment on three or more occasions in the recent past, and 30% had recently been hospitalised.[13] New treatment norms are now being implemented to reduce such deaths.[14] Children under five with severe malnutrition or persistent diarrhoea are now admitted to hospital. In addition, if dehydration brings a patient back within 24 hours of initial treatment, it is assumed that the mother is not using ORT correctly, and the child is hospitalised.

Because of the war and the health system's reduced capacity to provide services, a growing number of children in or near the war zones with diarrhoea do not receive any medical care or receive it too late. In war-affected areas, the number of visits for oral rehydration fell by more than

20% between 1985 and 1988. Because of the dangers and difficulties of travel, children in these areas are brought for treatment later, when dehydration is more severe, malnutrition is worse, and there is less chance of saving the child's life.

Poorer access to health facilities and a deterioration in living conditions have led to a sharp decline in the number of children hospitalised for diarrhoea and an alarming rise in the death rate among those who are hospitalised. Between 1983 and 1986 admissions to a hospital for diarrhoea declined 29% nationally, while the case fatality rate rose 79% (see Appendix 5). From 1983 to 1986 the reported number of deaths due to diarrhoea rose by 20% in hospitals and 10% outside hospitals. While the 1986 data are affected by improved reporting, and the reported number of deaths was still lower than in 1980, the indication was that diarrhoea-related mortality was on the increase.

The use of ORS packets as the mainstay of treatment has been heavily debated. Critics argue that parents should be encouraged to use a home-made solution of salt and sugar since these ingredients are more widely available than packets of ORS. Such home solutions are already the mainstay of treatment in isolated areas and war zones, where the ubiquitous Coca Cola bottle is used for mixing.

The use of ORS packets, it is argued, perpetuates dependency on the health service and imported goods. Defenders of ORS packets argue that their use has helped to give UROs the status of providers of medicine rather than 'merely' educational centres. In addition, health volunteers in rural areas gain additional status and credibility by having packets of ORS to distribute.

Over-emphasis on ORS packets, according to some health educators, has been associated with an approach which has been "insufficient, technocratic, and lacking in creativity".[15] ORS packets have been regarded as a cure-all, making it difficult for health education to "intervene effectively to change popular values and practices". Further, the use of ORS packets may result in children with chronic diarrhoea, associated respiratory infections, and serious nutritional deficiencies not receiving the necessary attention and treatment from doctors.

Diarrhoea is still the number one killer disease of infants and young children. In the 1970s it accounted for about half of all deaths among children. It now accounts for about a third of these deaths. The Government's goal is to to halve diarrhoea mortality among under-five-year-olds by 1991, in spite of the decline in living standards since the mid-1980s.[16] This decline has perpetuated the conditions under which diarrhoea is most common and serious: lack of sanitation and clean water supplies, poor hygiene, sub-standard housing, poverty and poor nutrition. Fernando Silva, Director of 'La Mascota' Children's Hospital in Managua, reflected:[17]

"We've carried out massive immunisation programmes in the

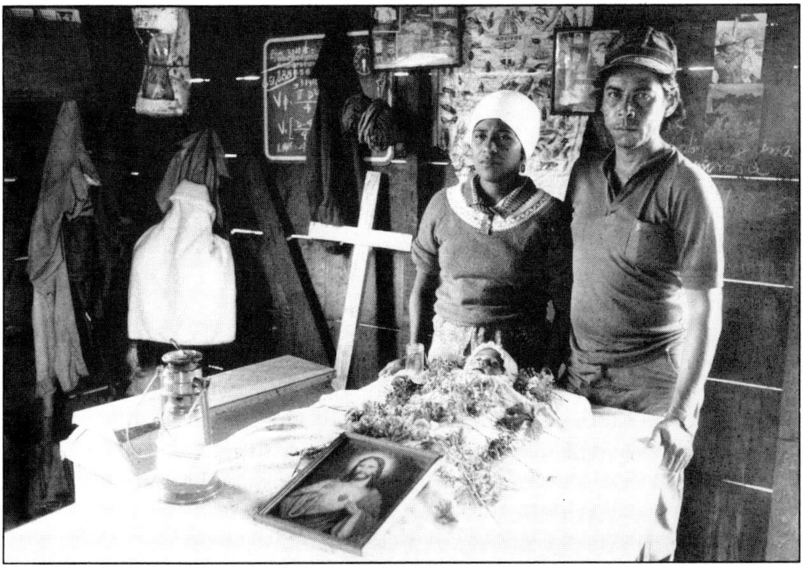

MIKE GOLDWATER

Diarrhoea is still the number one killer disease of infants and young children. This little girl died from diarrhoea-induced dehydration. She lived in a remote area of the Atlantic Coast, far from any health facilities.

community. There you have an action followed by an immediate reaction: an immunisation, which gives protection. So you have less measles, less whooping cough, less polio. But the only 'immunisation' against diarrhoea is for us to find a way out of poverty and underdevelopment."

Breast is best

Bottle-feeding is a leading contributor to infection, malnutrition and death among infants and young children in developing countries. A 1988 study in and around Managua found that children of illiterate mothers who were bottle-fed were three times more likely to be moderately or severely malnourished than children of illiterate mothers who were breastfed.

A large study in 1975 found that 58% of urban mothers and 69% of rural mothers breastfed for at least six months.[18] The practice of breastfeeding had declined rapidly during the 1970s, as baby milk manufacturers were marketing their products and their image of the 'modern' woman ever more aggressively. In 1978 a quarter of all mothers and a third of the mothers in Managua reported never having breastfed their last child.[19]

In 1980 MINSA launched a national campaign to promote breastfeeding and discourage bottle-feeding. Messages stressing the unique contribution which breast milk can make to a child's health and

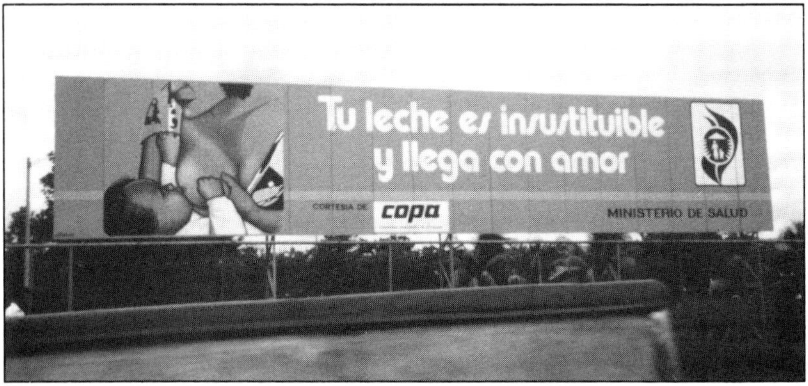
Tu leche es insustituible
y llega con amor
CORTESIA DE
copa
MINISTERIO DE SALUD

RICHARD GARFIELD

Roadside billboard: "Your milk is irreplaceable and comes with love".

well-being appeared on thousands of posters, billboards, and T-shirts. Hospital staff were instructed to encourage mothers to breastfeed, and 'rooming-in' of newborns was instituted to enable mothers to breastfeed on demand.[20] Bottles were banned from maternity wards, and milk banks set up for babies who, for whatever reason, were unable to breastfeed.[21] In 1981 a law was adopted based on the International Code of Marketing of Breast Milk Substitutes in order to curb the marketing practices of infant formula manufacturers. The Labour Code was also amended to allow women workers 12 weeks' maternity leave and to give mothers two half-hour breastfeeding breaks at the work place.

The campaign had to tread a thin line between openness and modesty. In 1980 the Government had banned the use of advertising which used women's bodies to promote the sales of commercial products. At the same time, the breastfeeding campaign showed images of plump, well-filled breasts, usually attached to the mouth of contented babies, on roadside billboards, T-shirts and posters.

The campaign seemed to have a good effect in Managua, where a survey in 1982 found that the percentage of mothers giving breast milk exclusively for the first four months rose from 26% to 50%.[22] This progress was short-lived. A similar survey in 1988 showed that more than half the mothers stopped giving the breast by the child's third month and only a quarter were still breastfeeding at six months.[23] One nurse observed, "They leave the hospital breastfeeding but have a bottle in their hand before they get on the bus to go home."

The problem is cultural, social and economic. About 70% of households are headed by women, many of whom are food vendors or market traders. For these women, breastfeeding at work is usually impractical. Women employed as domestic servants or in factories, hospitals or offices have the legal right to maternity leave and breastfeeding breaks at work; but without day-care facilities, and in the present harsh economic climate, these rights are often forgotten.

Many women who intend to breastfeed for months start bottle-feeding after just a few weeks. Why do so many stop? "I didn't have enough milk", "The baby wasn't satisfied", "The baby didn't want it" and "My doctor advised against it" are common responses. They are the result of both pervasive media images of the 'modern' woman, and the difficulty of maintaining mixed breast and bottle-feeding. They are also due to the failure of health workers to back up the breastfeeding campaign with appropriate counselling and advice.

The Government itself has not acted consistently. Until 1986 the Ministry of Social Welfare (INSSBI) provided infant formula to all new mothers at subsidised prices. MINSA has distributed bottles and infant formula to mothers through health posts and centres. In 1986, when baby bottles were so scarce they reached a black market price equal to a woman's weekly salary, the Government appealed to the international community for 50,000 new bottles. These were rushed from Italy and put onto the market in record time. Health Minister Tellez explained the dilemma:

"We have a culture of medicine-taking and milk supplementation. We have tried to eliminate imports of infant formula for economic reasons, but this created political problems. Working people want powdered milk, but we are working with half the dollars we had in 1983, and they must be prioritised for truly urgent imports, such as those for surgery."

"If you had only one egg..."

"If you had only one egg in the house, who would you give it to?" asked nutritionist Rosario Sandino, speaking to a group of expectant mothers at Velez Pais hospital in 1986. "Would you give it to your child, who is growing and needs it to build strong bones and muscle? To your husband, who works long hours and always comes home tired and hungry? Or would you eat it yourself to provide the nutrition you need to breastfeed your new baby?"

Every member of her audience agreed that the man should get the egg. After all, he was the one who brought home most of the money. If he fell ill or left the family, there would be even more days with only one egg. Rosario argued in favour of giving the egg to a child, or to the mother herself, but the women refused to budge. Each had faced this dilemma at some time. They were already used to having children who were small for their age.

Before 1979 more than half the under-five population suffered from some degree of malnutrition. During the first year of the revolution INSSBI distributed emergency rations via health and social welfare facilities.

In 1981 the Government stopped distributing rations routinely and began distributing food to families in need. INSSBI also distributed food

Fig. 9.2

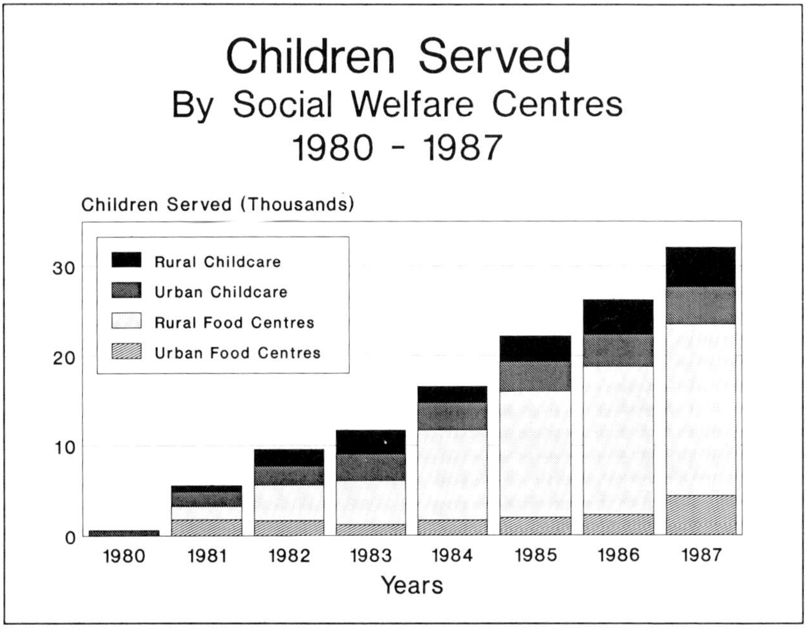

The number of children served by social welfare centres rose steadily through the 1980s.

via an expanding network of children's day-care centres. By 1988 about 38,000 children were attending 190 centres on cooperatives and state farms, and also in urban areas.[24] (see Figure 9.2) In rural areas the centres often consist of a wooden shelter with a thatch roof, a dirt floor and no walls. Food is cooked in great iron pots and served on plastic plates. If there is no cutlery, fingers are used. Despite poor physical conditions and a chronic shortage of staff and supplies, the centres are a great advance over the nine nurseries (eight of which were private) which existed before 1979. They are extremely popular with working mothers:

"If there was no day-care centre in our cooperative," said one mother, "I'd have to take my two young children with me into the fields. The only shelter there is under the trees or bushes. If it rains they get wet. They play in the soil and get dirty. But in the centre they get food and clothes, and books to read. They draw pictures. They're happy there, and I'm happy too."

The day-care centres have helped protect the health of tens of thousands of young children of low-income families. But they cater for only a small proportion of pre-school children, mainly in rural areas. Many malnourished children, especially in towns and cities, have no

Fig. 9.3

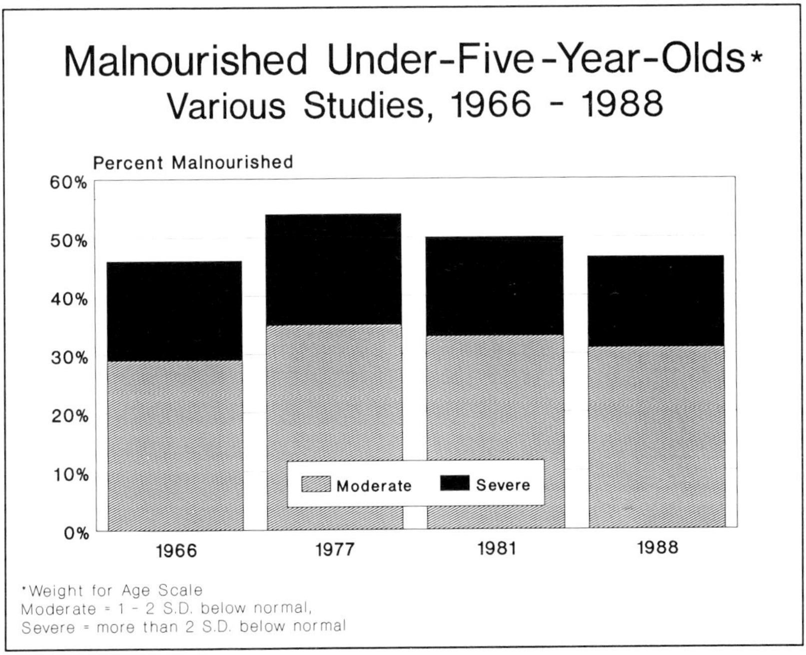

Malnutrition appears to have declined only slightly during the last 30 years.

local day-care centre to attend. Social worker Patricia Alfonso helped to organise a door-to-door survey by community volunteers in Ciudad Sandino in July 1988. The survey identified 539 malnourished children:

"These are the kids who at one year of age only weigh ten pounds. They are kept hidden, out of sight. The children's feeding centre is an initial effort to do something, but we know that this doesn't reach much of the population who need help."

With the economic crisis and the war, malnutrition among under-fives has again become widespread and nutritional rehabilitation units in hospitals are again full. Overall, there has been a modest decline in the proportion of moderately or severely malnourished children since the 1960s (see Figure 9.3) but 10% to 15% of babies born in hospitals still weigh less than 2,500 grams.[25]

Malnutrition is beyond the control of the curative health system. It is determined largely by factors such as the parents' education and income, the physical environment, the availability of food in sufficient quantity and quality, and overall economic conditions[26] (see Chapter 13). The *Contra* war and the country's economic decline since the mid-1980s have combined to perpetuate widespread malnutrition among children.[27]

Fig. 9.4

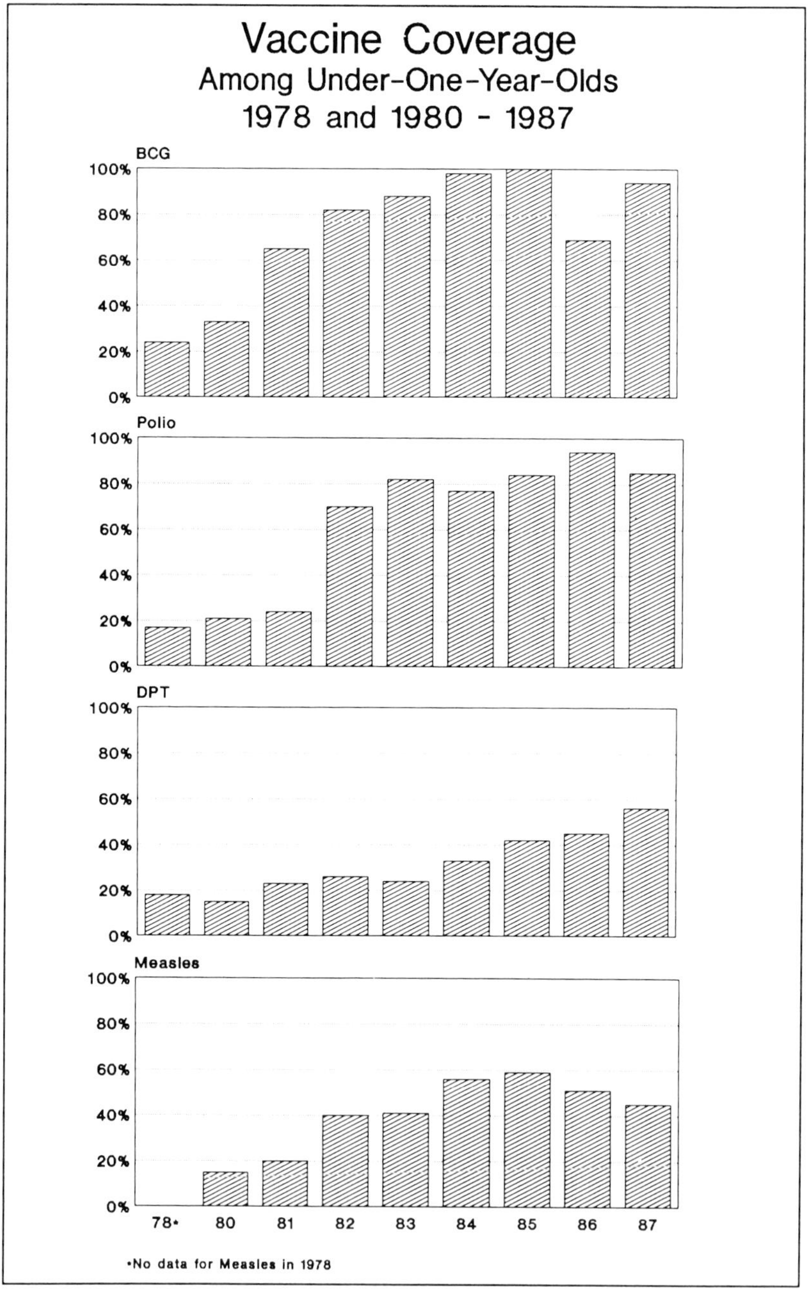
Vaccine Coverage
Among Under-One-Year-Olds
1978 and 1980 - 1987
BCG
Polio
DPT
Measles
100%
80%
60%
40%
20%
0%
78•
80
81
82
83
84
85
86
87
•No data for Measles in 1978

Immunisation

Immunisation against the six major vaccine-preventable diseases of infancy and childhood has increased dramatically since 1980 (see Figure 9.4). While mass campaigns (see Chapter 5) helped boost polio and measles coverage, routine immunisation at health clinics has also increased from year to year.

BCG coverage is now almost universal. It is carried out as part of the medical check-up which almost all babies receive (whether born at home or in hospital) during their first months. Unfortunately, the vaccine provides only limited protection from tuberculosis.

The other major vaccines have to be given when a child is older and therefore no longer so easy to bring to the health post. They are, however, far more important as they provide excellent protection against deadly diseases. Diphtheria-pertussis-tetanus coverage has increased steadily to 57% and continues to rise. Immunisation against polio has been over 80% each year since 1983. Measles coverage, after reaching almost 60% in 1985, fell to just over 40% in 1987. Immunisation of pregnant women against tetanus (which protects newborn babies against infection) reached 40% in 1986.

The impact of improved immunisation coverage on child health has been considerable. Cases of measles fell from about 1,000 a year during the 1970s to only 80 in 1984. Tetanus deaths (the great majority among newborns) fell from about 240 annually before 1979 to around 50 in the mid-1980s (see Chapter 7). No cases of polio were reported between 1982 and 1988.

The war

Among those under 15 years of age, there have been 455 war-related deaths, 691 kidnappings, and 1,542 war-induced injuries. Some 1,200 children suffer long-term disabilities as a result of the war.[28] These include 200 spinal cord injuries, 100 burn victims, and 290 amputations.[29] More than 10,000 children have lost a father or mother, and 600 children have lost both parents in the war. An estimated 180,000 children have been forced to leave their homes to seek safety (see Figure 9.5).

Child health programmes have been disrupted in the war zones. In the community of Patastillal near Jinotega, for example, immunisation stopped completely after *Contra* troops murdered one of two local health volunteers in late 1986. It was not until April 1988, during a cease-fire, that a health team was able to vaccinate children and pregnant women. Local residents also took the opportunity to rebuild the school and health

< Fig. 9.4 – Vaccine coverage among under-one-year-olds improved in the 1980s but is still inadequate for measles and diptheria-pertussis-tetanus vaccine. These MINSA estimates are calculated at the beginning of each year before initiating vaccination campaigns.

Fig. 9.5

Number of Nicaraguans Under Age 17 Affected by the War, 1988

	Nicaragua	Honduras	Costa Rica
Living in the War Zone	130,000		
Living in the Periphery of the War Zone	225,000		
Displaced from War Zone, living in Nicaragua	160,000		
Refugees Outside Nicaragua:			
In Camps		13,000	4,000
Out of Camps		14,000	24,000
Returned Refugees	12,000		

Source: CARE, *Children's survival assistance programme needs assessment team field report: Nicaragua*, New York: CARE, 1988.

clinic, both of which had been destroyed by the *Contras*. A new health volunteer also came forward for training.

Changes in mortality rates

Despite the *Contra* war and declining living standards, a Nicaraguan child's chances of survival have improved dramatically since 1979. Between 1978 and 1983, the infant mortality rate fell by about a third (see Figure 9.6). (The actual decline depends on the quality of estimates of mortality at present and assumptions about mortality levels prior to the revolution. Mortality rate estimates for 1978 vary from a low of 90 to a high of 120 per 1,000 live births. A review of demographic studies by Behm suggest that the lower figure is more accurate.[30])

Infant mortality had declined by about two deaths per 1,000 births per year during the 1960s and 1970s. The accelerated decline during the early 1980s, averaging about four per 1,000 per year, was striking. Most of this dramatic decline can be traced to three specific actions: diarrhoea treatment and prevention, immunisation against measles, and improved literacy rates among mothers. Rapid urbanisation is an additional factor associated with the acceleration of the decline.

Nicaragua and Honduras have long had similar population, economic and mortality dynamics. A comparison of infant deaths registered by cause during 1985/86 reveals the near-disappearance of deaths from

Fig. 9.6

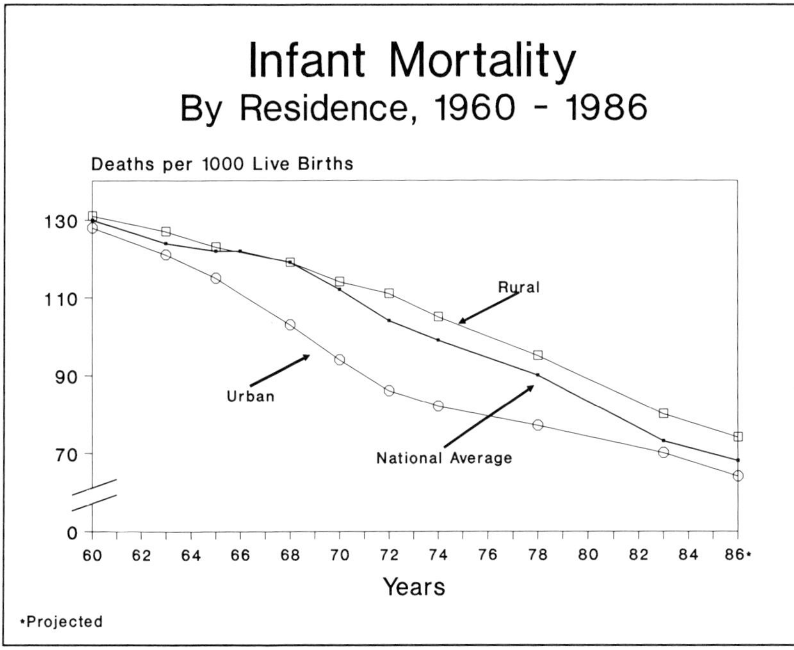

Estimated infant mortality rates declined earlier and more rapidly in urban areas. The accelerated decline during the early 1980s is associated with a narrowing of the gap between urban and rural mortality rates and the increased urbanisation of the country.

vaccine-preventable diseases in Nicaragua (see Figure 9.7). Deaths from diarrhoea and respiratory disease were also lower. In both countries, respiratory and diarrhoeal diseases remain the main preventable causes of infant deaths. It is likely that the rates of perinatal deaths in Nicaragua and Honduras are similar; data in Figure 9.7 probably differ because of the higher rate of hospitalisation (and therefore greater likelihood of registration) of infants in Nicaragua.

The single greatest influence on infant mortality appears to be improved literacy among mothers. Although infant mortality declined in each decade since the 1960s at each level of mother's schooling, a dramatic drop followed the literacy crusade of 1980 (see Figure 9.8). Among illiterate mothers in 1982/83, 95 of every 1,000 newborns died before completing 12 months. Among mothers who were literate but had not attended school, only 75 per 1,000 died. Thus, when 90% of mothers-to-be without schooling became literate in 1980, the deaths of more than 1,000 babies each year were prevented. This alone accounted for a decline in infant mortality of about 10% and represents close to a fifth of

Fig. 9.7

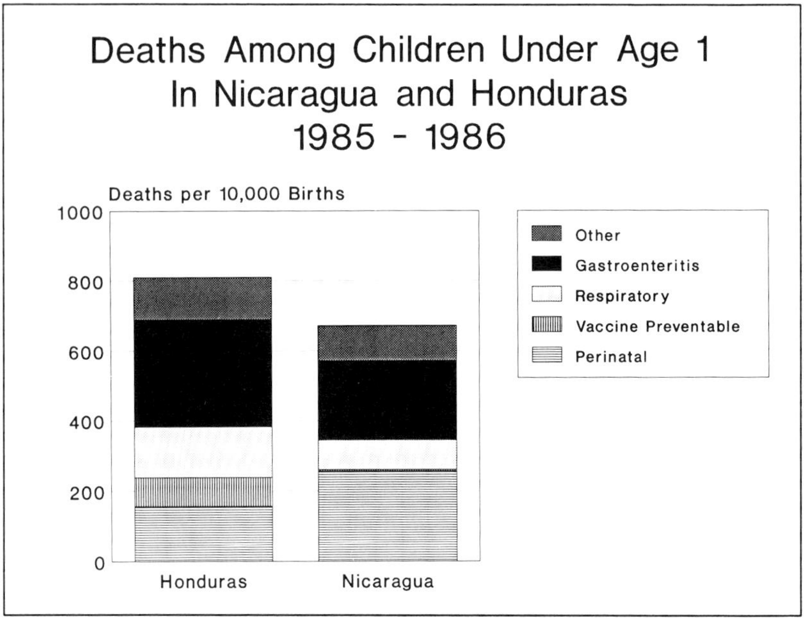

Infant mortality rates in Nicaragua are notably lower than those for Honduras for causes which respond to the major child health programmes in Nicaragua. These programmes include vaccination for vaccine-preventable diseases, oral rehydration for diarrhoea and antibiotic treatment for respiratory infections.

the total infant mortality decline from 1978 to 1983.

Infant mortality has fallen faster in rural than in urban areas (see Figure 9.6). This may be due to the Government's efforts to target social and economic development programmes on the rural poor as well as increased maternal literacy. However, mortality is still about 50% greater in rural areas.

The affluent had experienced infant mortality rates which were one-fourth those of the poor during the 1970s. While the magnitude of this difference has narrowed by half in Nicaragua, it remains broad in most of the rest of Central America. This narrowing appears to result from improved living conditions for the poor (at least until 1985).

Registered death rates for children aged one to four in Nicaragua during 1985/86 can be compared with data for 1975/76. During that ten-year period, deaths from vaccine-preventable diseases and diarrhoea declined precipitously (see Figure 9.9). Respiratory diseases declined slightly among one to four-year-olds, while deaths from violence increased.

Fig. 9.8

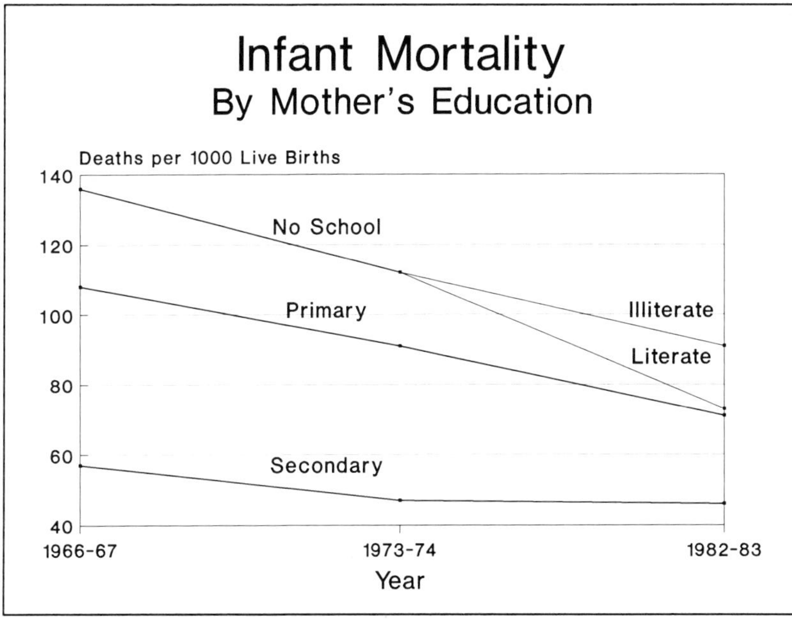

Declines in the infant mortality rate are associated in recent years with higher educational levels of the mother. It appears that maternal literacy alone is responsible for the greatest reduction in risk of infant death.

Mortality among this age group declined more slowly between 1978 and 1987, falling by about 25%.[31] This decline is half as great as the decline among infants. This is probably because infant mortality responds well to targeted medical and social interventions, while mortality among one to four-year-olds responds more to the overall living conditions.

These improvements still leave a great deal to be done. Of the more than 100,000 children born in Nicaragua each year, approximately 10,000 die before the age of five. About 6,000 die in their first year and 4,000 die in the next four years. Only one in every five Nicaraguans is under five years of age, but 42% of all estimated deaths occur in this age group.[32]

Large geographic disparities also still exist. In the poorest regions infant mortality is about twice as high as in the most affluent regions.[33] Although the level of the mother's education is closely associated with risk of death during the first five years, even children of illiterate mothers in the Department of Managua had a better chance than the children of mothers who graduated from secondary school in outlying regions.

Even more disturbing is the fact that, since the mid-1980s, the downward curve in infant deaths has almost flattened out (see Figure 9.6).

Fig. 9.9

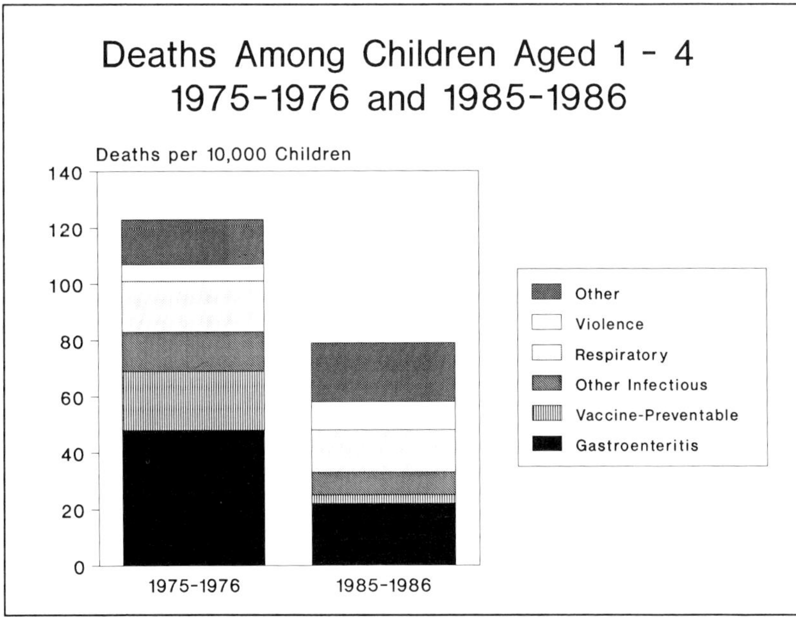

Over the span of a decade, deaths from diarrhoea and vaccine-preventable diseases among one to four-year-old children were considerably reduced. Deaths from violent causes, however, increased.

In 1987 the infant mortality rate in Nicaragua was estimated at about 65 per 1,000 births. This rate was similar to those for El Salvador, Guatemala and Honduras, and much higher than that for Costa Rica.[34]

Yet such high rates of infant and child death are not inevitable, even in a country beset by war and a severe economic crisis. Most infant and child deaths are still due to several preventable diseases. The Latin American Demographic Centre (CELADE) projects that at least 5,500 deaths among under-five-year-olds could be prevented through improved nutrition, diarrhoea control, and the prompt treatment of respiratory infections.[35]

'Defending the lives of children'

Against this background MINSA launched the 'Campaign to Defend the Lives of Children' on 6 August 1988. In a speech that day emphasising the Government's intention to make the campaign a major national priority, President Ortega called on "all political parties, churches, and people's organisations to join together to combat infant mortality".

The campaign aims to cut infant deaths by promoting diarrhoea control, immunisation, breastfeeding, birth spacing, maternal care, treatment of respiratory infections and improved nutrition.[36] The campaign has a strong inter-sectorial approach, with other government ministries including Education, Transport and Social Welfare prominently involved. At the community level, organisations such as the Sandinista Defence Committees, trade unions, and youth, student, and women's organisations have been assigned leading roles. But the Government is also seeking support from sections of the community which have often been hostile to the revolution — such as business leaders and the hierarchy of the Roman Catholic Church. Said programme coordinator Carolina Siu:

"Business groups and conservative sectors of the church cannot oppose us in this effort. Now they are on the spot, just like us. MINSA is not running this campaign. The Ministry is simply the technical secretary for a broad national crusade to save children's lives."

Local government is also involved. Plans to improve water and waste disposal are being developed locally under each mayor's direction. Community organisations are being called on to help identify malnourished children and provide them with supplementary food, depending on local resources. Cooperatives and state farms, for example, are encouraged to set aside a cow or chickens in order to provide a secure supply of milk or eggs to children in need. At a national meeting of the farmers' organisation (UNAG), male delegates were sceptical of this provision. Female leaders pushed through a resolution supporting the MINSA request and promised to see that it gets carried out.

The campaign is the major planned programme to be undertaken by MINSA during the last years of the 1980s. Although it is the focus of many Ministry activities, it was launched with few new resources and has been implemented as the health budget and staff was reduced by 30%. Its chances of success depend in large part on the international aid it attracts. The diarrhoea control programme, for example, will require large investments in improved water supplies and sanitation facilities — investments which are well beyond the capacity of the Government to provide.

Unlike past health programmes, which targeted whole sectors of the population, the 'Campaign to Defend the Lives of Children' is focusing its limited resources on those groups in greatest need. Nutritional programmes in the work place, for example, are targeted on pregnant women. Special efforts are also being made by health workers and community groups to reach mothers-to-be who are illiterate (15% of the total), geographically isolated (5%), or at high risk because they are either under 20 (21%) or over 40 years old (2%).[37]

The potential for improving the health of children appears to be great. Hospitals and health centres were directed to review their records and identify patterns associated with high infant death rates when the campaign began. It was found in Berta Calderon Hospital, for example, that most deaths among newborns occurred late at night or in the early morning, when no paediatric specialists are present. In the second half of 1988, when at least one neonatologist was put on duty in the hospital at all times, the death rate was cut by half.

Yet much of the potential for health promotion has hardly been explored.[38] Nutritional education, growth monitoring, and rooming-in for breastfeeding, for example, are only occasionally carried out. These preventive actions would bring enormous benefit to vulnerable children, but their appeal to doctors with a curative orientation is limited.

The campaign's main focus, nonetheless, is on parental education, to help parents understand what they can do to protect and promote their children's health. According to campaign leader Dr. Ivan Tercero, "We need to do three things for child health: improve water and sanitation, provide better nutrition, and carry out more education. We hardly have the funds even to start doing the first two, but improved health education and use of our resources is within our reach."

Specific targets have been set and local leaders are using them to monitor progress. For immunisation, the goal is to reach at least 80% of the target population for each of the six main vaccine-preventable childhood diseases. One hundred percent coverage is expected in many parts of the country. Ironically, Managua is one of the regions plagued by low coverage. While polio vaccine coverage was estimated at 82% nationally for 1988, it was only 74% in Managua. For prenatal care, the goal is for at least 75% of all pregnant women to have at least three check-ups during pregnancy.

For a country beset by war, economic deterioration and natural disasters, the campaign is extremely ambitious. There are no precedents in the developing world for such a dramatic reduction in infant mortality under similar conditions. Many believe that the campaign can be regarded as successful if all it does is to prevent infant mortality from rising.

Yet one lesson of recent years in Nicaragua is that well-designed health programmes, targeted on specific groups, and implemented with the participation of a wide cross-section of the community, can achieve impressive results. The successes of the immunisation and malaria programmes are the most obvious examples. If the new campaign focuses on educating and involving the community rather than perpetuating dependency on doctors, hospitals and medicines, it may succeed. But the campaign may have an even wider impact. Says Programme Director Carolina Siu:

"The war has left us a divided society. We hope this campaign can be a point of departure from which to rebuild our society, to strengthen the social fabric. If effective, this campaign will help unite all of Nicaragua, like the Literacy Crusade did in 1980."

Chapter 10: Health Professionals

"The state will establish mechanisms to involve health professionals in the formulation and implementation of the health plan."
(*Proclamation of the Government of National Reconstruction,* 18 July 1979.)

"If it weren't for my private practice I wouldn't stay in this country."
(an anonymous doctor)

From the moment they came to power the Sandinistas were haunted by the fear of a mass exodus of doctors. Recent precedents in other Latin American countries were hardly reassuring. In Cuba, the emigration of about half the country's doctors within three years of the revolution in 1959 destabilised the country's health and political systems.[1] In Chile, medical opposition frustrated reforms initiated by Salvador Allende's socialist Government, helping to create favourable conditions for the right-wing coup of 1973.[2] Sandinista leaders feared a similar 'fight or flight' reaction in their country. The issue was as much political as medical. Doctors were prominent members of the middle class. They would need to be won over for the Sandinistas to succeed in their stated intention of developing a 'pluralist' society and a 'mixed' economy.

Doctors did begin leaving the country, but in a trickle rather than a flood. There were three main reasons why the much-feared mass exodus failed to occur. First, opportunities to work in the United States were far more restricted in 1979 than they had been in 1959. Second, as one of the inheritances of the Somoza era, many doctors trained in Nicaragua did not meet the technical standards required by other countries. And third, the revolutionary Government made herculean efforts to satisfy the doctors. First among these efforts was the appointment of a non-political neurosurgeon, widely respected in medical circles, as the first Minister of Health. Doctors believed, with good reason, that the Government would respect their professional integrity.

The trickle of doctors out of the country was offset by an influx of foreign health professionals, who numbered about 800 in the peak year of 1982. Most of the *internacionalistas* came from Western Europe and

Latin America, especially Mexico and Cuba; some also came from the United States. Most provided services to populations in rural areas never previously reached by modern health care. Dozens of Nicaraguan doctors who favoured the overthrow of Somoza also returned to the country immediately after the dictator was deposed.[3]

The absence of Nicaraguan doctors was most notable in specialties including anaesthesia, ophthalmology and internal medicine. Later, when the *Contra* war became more widespread, rehabilitation and neurosurgery were the specialties in greatest shortage. In a small country, where there are normally only two or three specialists in particular areas of medicine, the loss of even one can be serious. The lack of specialists was felt most acutely in the Medical School in Leon, where teaching in some subject areas had to be suspended for lack of qualified staff.

Opposition political groups seized upon the issue of foreign health workers. *La Prensa* newspaper published inflammatory stories suggesting that foreign doctors were unqualified to practise medicine in their own countries, were covert military personnel rather than health professionals, and spread venereal diseases due to their poor health and immoral behaviour.[4] Cuban doctors were a particular target of rumour, innuendo and defamation. None of the accusations were justified. Many Cubans doctors have served in isolated rural areas and war zones where national physicians preferred not to venture.

The biggest surge in the numbers of departing doctors occurred in 1983, when the *Contra* war escalated and a military draft was initiated. In the first half of 1983 about 200 doctors (including 88 specialists) left the country.[5] Consequently, some urban neighbourhoods and rural communities which had grown used to having a doctor suddenly found themselves without one. By the end of 1986, 646 doctors, close to half of all working in the country before 1979, had left.[6] Their departure deprived the health system of valuable medical expertise. On the other hand, moderate Sandinista policies had minimised the impact of this brain drain. The loss had been gradual and had not destabilised the political system. And in the meantime, hundreds of newly trained doctors had begun to work (see Figure 10.1).

The continued emigration of physicians was nonetheless a cause for concern. Especially alarming was the realisation that specialists trained since 1979 were also leaving. Of the 29 obstetrics-gynaecology specialists working in the country in 1985, 22 had left by 1988. The pro-Sandinista newspaper *El Nuevo Diario* appealed to the Government to try to reduce medical emigration:[7]

"A policy of encouragement would include sufficient salaries and technical facilities to carry out their work efficiently, and other actions that the health authorities can well determine. This would not be creating a privileged sector of professionals, but would respond to the objective reality of a country which has a grave and chronic shortage of doctors,

Fig. 10.1

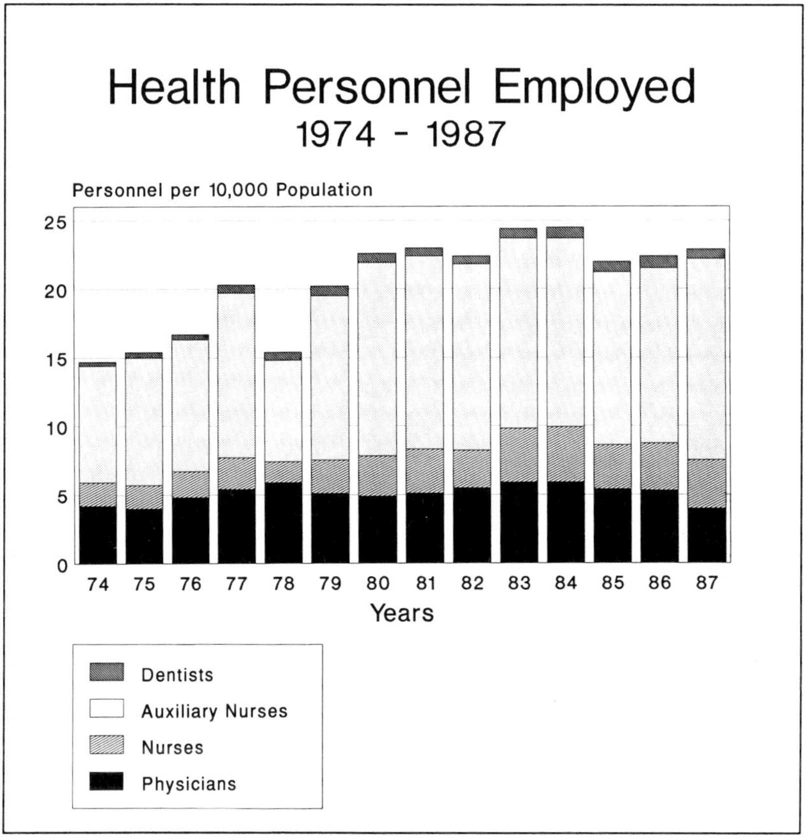

A rapid rise in the number of health workers employed has only moderately exceeded the rate of population growth.

and which cannot afford the luxury of sitting by passively while doctors continue to leave."

Nubia Herrera, a prominent nursing leader, took a different view:

"If half the doctors leave but the ones who stay are with the revolution, we'll be OK. The problem now is that half the doctors are dragging their feet and weakening the revolution's health programmes."

The white coat empire

Doctors leave the country for financial, professional and social reasons. A dramatic fall in real income and the economic chaos caused by rampant inflation have been key factors. Many also resent government attempts at regulation and a loss of status in today's more egalitarian society.

Regulation of medical practice was sorely needed. During the Somoza regime there was no system even for registering physicians. Nor were there any criteria for official recognition of specialists: doctors would simply advertise themselves in the press as 'paediatric haematologists' or 'renal surgeons' without any specific qualifications. In addition, many doctors exploited the public health service by drawing government salaries while spending most of their time in private practice. Some doctors worked only a few hours a day in public clinics but were paid for as many as 20 hours of work. The total number of reimbursed medical hours even surpassed the physical capacities of some of the most notorious clinics.

In 1980 the Government proposed a bill to establish government regulation of medical practice. This was fiercely opposed by the medical establishment, who organised a one-day walk-out from hospitals in protest at what they regarded as government interference in their professional affairs.[8] The heavily political character of the medical opposition, including threats of mass emigration to Miami, had a chilling effect on relations between doctors' leaders and the Government. A Health Ministry official said angrily: "These people live in a dream world. They say that if we pressure them they will go to the US where they can pursue their profession freely. But in the US there is far more regulation and control over medical practice than has been proposed here."

Representatives of the *Colegio de Medicos* took part in redrafting the bill, and some of its provisions were watered down. Only in 1983 did it finally become law.[9] Yet the precedent set was extremely important. For the first time, the medical establishment was obliged to accept the right of the government to regulate their professional practice. As a result, doctors receiving a salary were required to increase their scheduled public practice to at least six hours a day and to fulfil their contracted time. Salaries for public service at each professional level were standardised and a maximum salary level established. The one-year social service requirement for medical graduates was extended to two years, greatly increasing the number of doctors working in rural areas.

Changes in regulation and practice were not well received by all members of the medical profession. An anonymous letter writer to *La Prensa* on 12 June 1985 complained:[10]

"Today the doctor has a lower social rank. Doctors come mainly from the middle class and aspire to a better standard of living. Today doctors feel limited or even worse, pushed down the social ladder. It is not uncommon to hear doctors complain that in hospitals they are treated as though they were plumbers or air conditioner repairmen. This style of egalitarianism is a fallacy, because in all industrialised countries of the East and West, doctors have certain social privileges."

Yet the influence and prestige of the medical profession remains enormous. One group of doctors has concentrated on strengthening the formal organs of professional influence, the powerful *Colegio de Medicos* and *Federacion de Sociedades Medicas.* These associations are now better organised and more influential than before the revolution. A second, smaller group of left-of-centre doctors is active in the health workers' union FETSALUD. A third group has avoided all forms of organisation, any of which they view as open to government manipulation. In their various ways, these three groups are well-placed to influence the political process. In 1985, for example, when the Government formed a commission to try to standardise the anarchic system of doctors' fees in private practice, the organised opposition of the medical profession led to abandonment of the idea.[11] There are, however, important new limits to the political power of organised medicine. When doctors in Managua went on strike in August 1988, the Health Minister soon got them back to work by threatening to replace them all with Cubans.

Many aspects of medical practice still remain lax. When the nurse in charge of the health post in San Lorenzo, Boaco department, moved to Managua in 1987, she was replaced by a social service doctor straight out of medical school. Within a few weeks what had been an exemplary rural health service began to disintegrate. The young doctor spent only three days per week in San Lorenzo, devoting the rest of his time to establishing a lucrative private practice three hours away in Managua. Worse still, he charged for medical consultations in the health post.

Since his was the only service available, the local people had little choice but to pay him or go without care. When they finally complained to the regional health authorities and asked for another doctor to be sent in his place, visits to the post had so declined that San Lorenzo could no longer be considered a high priority area. The people would have to wait until more new doctors graduated. Meanwhile, someone scrawled the people's feelings on the wall of the health post: "Too bad doctors do social service rather than compulsory army service on the war front...."

Private medicine

In 1979 it was thought that medicine would eventually be completely socialised. According to Dr. Antonio Jarquin, one of the early architects of the system, "It was impossible to do this with the resources we had. [For the time being] private medicine would be like a safety valve."[12] In 1989, however, about 90% of doctors have private practices. Only in isolated areas, where foreign volunteers and recent Nicaraguan medical graduates work, is private medicine absent. Following two years of social service, doctors are free to go private. This issue was raised during debates in the National Assembly during 1986 on a new national constitution. Sandinista delegates, including several doctors, denounced private medicine as an exploitation of the people, while representatives of other parties defended the right of doctors to exercise their professional skills outside the state health system.

The constitution, as finally approved, was a compromise, referring only to the area upon which most delegates agreed, namely, that it is the responsibility of the government to ensure that the health needs of the population are provided for. The right of medical professionals to practise privately is not explicitly recognised, but neither is it denied.

As the *Contra* war and the economic crisis worsened, doctors became increasingly dependent on their private practices. According to Dr. Leonel Arguello, Head of Epidemiology in MINSA:

"Attitudes toward private practice have changed a lot. We thought that if health could be considered a right, private care would have to be eliminated. At first it was regarded as being only for the ethically weak or politically uncommitted. But theory and practice weren't the same. Progressive doctors started leaving MINSA in order to make ends meet. Now, many revolutionaries have gone into private practice on a part-time basis, and no-one accuses them of backsliding. It is, in fact, the only realistic option available."

In a few hours of private medical practice a doctor can earn the equivalent of a month's salary in the public health system. This combination of public service and private enterprise is also carried out by many nurses and other health professionals, albeit at lower levels of remuneration.

In Managua, typically, private medicine is practised at an office in a clinic or attached to the home. In small towns it may be an office, complete with an elaborate sign, off the town square. Those who use private care the most are middle-class people, market traders, and government employees. Some of the best care is private, as well as some of the worst.

Work in the public system has some important advantages. It offers far greater opportunities to utilise modern medical equipment and interact with other professionals. Another benefit is easier access to basic commodities such as rice and soap, and imported goods such as cars. Most physicians, including those trained since the revolution, work six hours a day in public medicine and two to four hours a day in their private practices. Others, however, work only in private practice through an office or private hospital.

Private practice is not likely to disappear. Since 1988 all new health centres built by MINSA have public and private offices under the same roof. In 1989 a private ward was established in a public hospital in Jinotepe and another in Managua.[13] In this way, MINSA hopes to generate additional operating funds and persuade newly trained physicians to remain in the country. Nonetheless, the Government is nervous about the uncontrolled growth of private medicine. A *La Prensa* editorial mocked this concern by suggesting that MINSA believes "there are more clinics in Managua than food shops in the *barrios*."[14]

Whatever its drawbacks, private care does help meet the social aspirations of doctors and provides treatment which affluent patients prefer. It also absorbs surplus money which is difficult to spend because of the lack of luxury goods for sale. In this way, both doctors and their better-off patients are able to maintain a semblance of middle-class life despite the rampant inflation and chronic shortages which beset the country.

Training doctors

In 1979 there was one doctor on average for every 2,100 people, but their distribution was highly skewed. In the major cities there was an average of 1,400 people per doctor, compared with 5,000 in the rest of the country. Admission to the one medical school, in the city of Leon, was tightly restricted. No more than 55 students were admitted each year. At this rate, a desirable doctor/patient ratio would never have been reached. The revolutionary Government therefore decided to train a large cadre of new doctors, at the rate of 500 per year. Professor Fabio Salamanca, former Dean of the Leon Medical School, explained:

"Many of us had participated in the revolution and were sympathetic to the Sandinistas. In the 1970s we had tried to make changes in the curriculum, to accept students from rural and poor backgrounds, and to

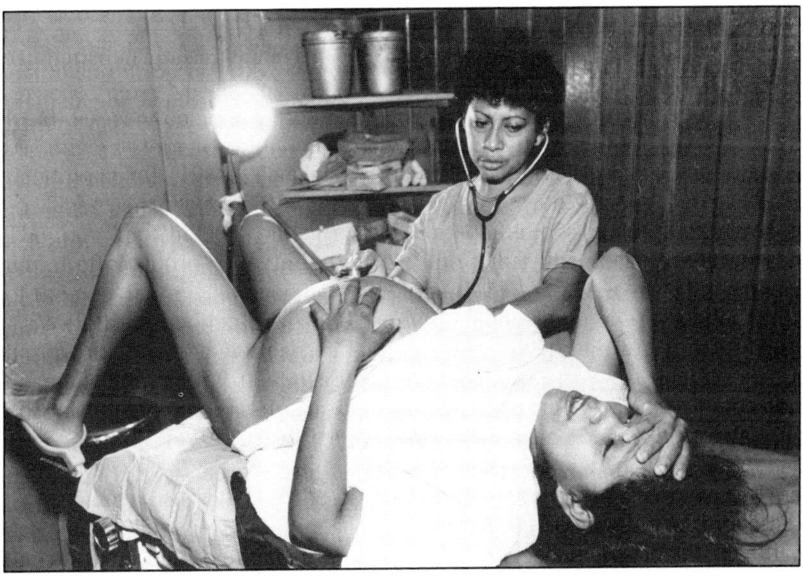

MIKE GOLDWATER

After graduating, all doctors work for two years in a 'social service' post. Recently graduated doctor cares for a woman in labour, in a hospital in the war zone.

make practical experience and independent thinking a priority. But our efforts were stopped by the directors of the school. When the Sandinistas came to power, we saw our opportunity to make important changes in the curriculum. But more importantly, we felt that it was necessary to produce more, to turn out more physicians as our contribution to the revolution."

A second medical school, in Managua, was started in 1981.[15] Five years later, 400 newly graduated doctors took up their social service posts. In the small auditorium of the surgical hospital in the northern town of La Trinidad, which only six months earlier had been attacked by *Contra* troops, sat 82 of these young physicians. They listened anxiously as health officials briefed them on the local situation. Their arrival would, at one stroke, double the number of doctors in the region. Their medical education, however, had differed in many important ways from that of their older colleagues.

What doctors learn

Nicaraguan medical education underwent extensive revision in the early 1980s.[16] The number of doctors in training rose ten-fold while classroom and laboratory supplies and space hardly changed. Most students only managed to see real text books in the library; they studied and worked from mimeographed notes which they bound into home-made texts. The clinical and teaching expertise of teachers prior to 1979 was limited. Following 1979, many of the best teachers either left the country or took leadership positions in MINSA. Gaps in clinical training became painfully apparent.

The revised medical curriculum emphasises disease prevention, participation in a health team, the role of the community in promoting good health, and the social roots of disease.[17] Social science courses have been added as well as courses in epidemiology, health administration and environmental health.

The major innovation of the new curriculum is the work-study programme. From their first week in medical school, students spend one day every week working in the community with patients and local organisations. Together with health volunteers, first-year students conduct community health surveys, including evaluation of the health status of families. They also administer vaccines, give educational talks and help link the community with local centres. This 'hands on' experience can have a strong effect on students. As one student said:

"When I first arrived in the community people began to ask me questions and I had no idea of the answers. So I came back to medical school and studied more."

In their second year students work with children in primary schools learning about growth monitoring, immunisation, health education and diarrhoeal disease control. During their third year they study nutrition, collect stool samples and inspect work sites. In the fourth year their course work focuses on occupational health, and they work in factories and health centres. In their fifth and final year, they work in health centres and hospitals and learn about maternal and child care.

In addition to their work-study programme, most students also spend two months a year working in special work brigades. Many staff and students help with the coffee or cotton harvest. Many also take part in health days (such as immunisation campaigns), or assist the health services during emergencies such as the aftermath of Hurricane Joan in October 1988. Some also serve as medical orderlies in militia and army units.[18] These 'mobilisations' can be enormously time-consuming. Denis Silva Torres, who in 1983 became the first medical student killed in the *Contra* war, had spent more time off-campus than on-campus during his training. Melvin Agurcia, who graduated in 1984, volunteered four times as a medical orderly in the army. His reasons were simple: "We future doctors should be motivated by pride in everything our people are doing to defend our sovereignty and independence."

But the loss of course time through mobilisations also contributed to a decline in the quality of clinical training. In 1985 a majority of all third-year students failed one or more clinical courses, and one-third had to repeat the entire academic year. A reassessment in 1986 led to important changes. Students can no longer volunteer for health campaigns, harvests, or service in the militia or army, except as part of a programme sponsored by the medical school. Although male students can perform military service, they are kept for only one academic year. The work-study programme has also been cut from 20% to 10% of course time, and basic sciences have been reintroduced in the first year of medical studies.

Efforts are being made to bring students from less affluent families into medicine. These efforts include a scholarship programme, a residential pre-medicine high school course organised at the medical school for rural students, and on-campus housing for medical students from outlying regions. Regional quotas also give students from outside Managua (60% of all students) a better chance to matriculate. According to Nubia Herrera, former Director of the Medical School Department of Preventive Medicine:

"These students are middle-class by local standards, but would be considered poor by Managua standards. Some of them do better than students from Managua, because many didn't suffer as much disruption in their secondary education as those from the city."

The proportion of female medical students has risen steadily since 1980 and in 1984 passed the 50% mark.

Surprisingly, many believe that preventive medicine and community health training are the weakest aspects of current medical education. There are several reasons for this. First, the schools are not run by MINSA but by the National Higher Education Council,[19] a group more interested in the development of expertise than in its application. Second, the best teachers of preventive medicine are no longer at the medical schools. Finally, the work-study programme has often exploited students for their labour, but has done little to encourage an interest in primary health care.

Training remains heavily oriented toward hospitals, and little classroom time is devoted to ambulatory or primary care. As a result, many new graduates are more prepared to prescribe medicines than to encourage breastfeeding, growth monitoring, or home-mixes for oral rehydration therapy, and are reluctant to work with traditional birth attendants. According to Dr. Ennio Cufino, formerly of the Managua office of UNICEF, "The only aspects of preventive medicine to gain respect among medical students are programmes like immunisations and malaria treatment which don't intrude upon the hospital-based, curative care system."

Nursing in crisis

Like medicine, nursing in Nicaragua was organised on a model 'made in the USA'.[20] Military and other nurses who accompanied the US Marines to Nicaragua early in this century introduced high standards of clinical education which were poorly suited to the needs of a developing country. Most Nicaraguan nurses were in fact auxiliaries, or aides, trained in courses of six to twelve months. Others were known as 'empiricals', with no formal training at all.[21]

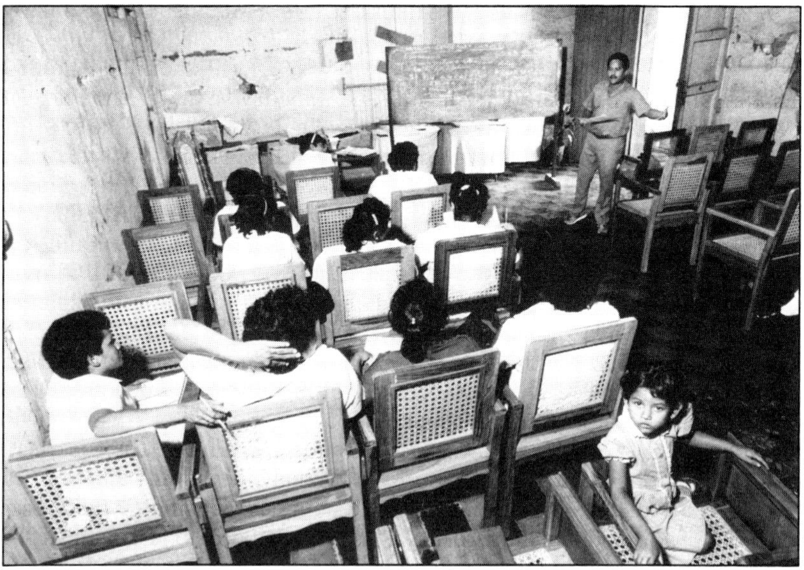

MIKE GOLDWATER

Nurses attend a refresher course on the treatment of malaria.

Fig. 10.2

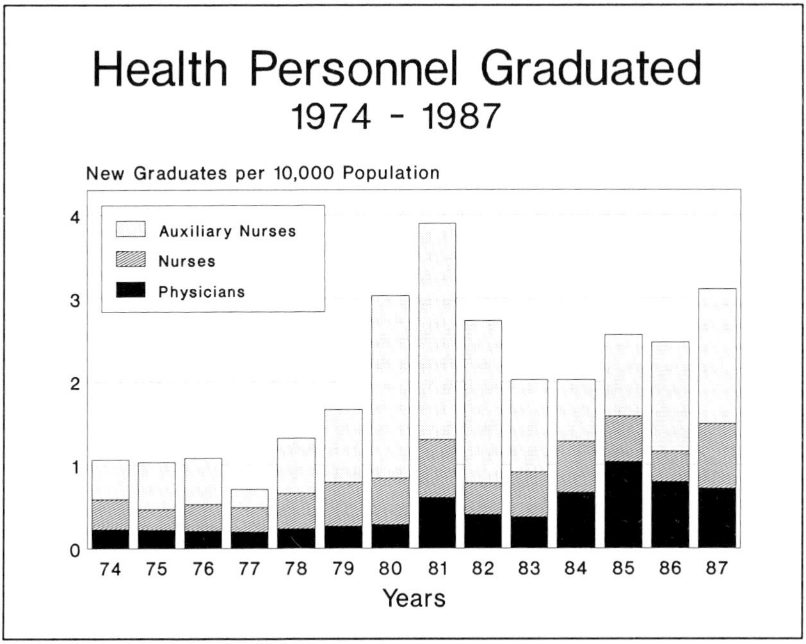

New auxiliary nurses trained in the first years of the revolution soon came into the work force, while new physicians only began to appear in 1984.

The Somoza regime feared the influence of nurses in politics, labour and health care issues even more that that of doctors. The regime tried hard to keep nurses divided. Professional responsibilities and salaries varied widely: the salaries of nurses in hospitals and clinics in Managua were about three times higher than those of nurses working in outlying areas. Responsibility for the training of nurses was something of a merry-go-round. When the North American director of the nursing school left in 1950, control was assumed in turn by a religious order, the Ministry of Health, the University, and then the Ministry of Health once more.

The revolution's new health programmes created an enormous need for more and better-trained nurses in primary care and more sophisticated hospital-based care.[22] The Government has trained large numbers of nursing auxiliaries: between 1980 and 1987 the number of nursing aides trained increased ten-fold. At the same time the numbers trained in a basic, three-year course increased five-fold (see Figure 10.2). This is still far from adequate, as about 8% of nurses leave the profession every year: some emigrate to the United States, but most find other work in the country because of dissatisfaction with pay and working conditions.

There is currently a more serious shortage of nurses than of doctors. In

Fig. 10.3

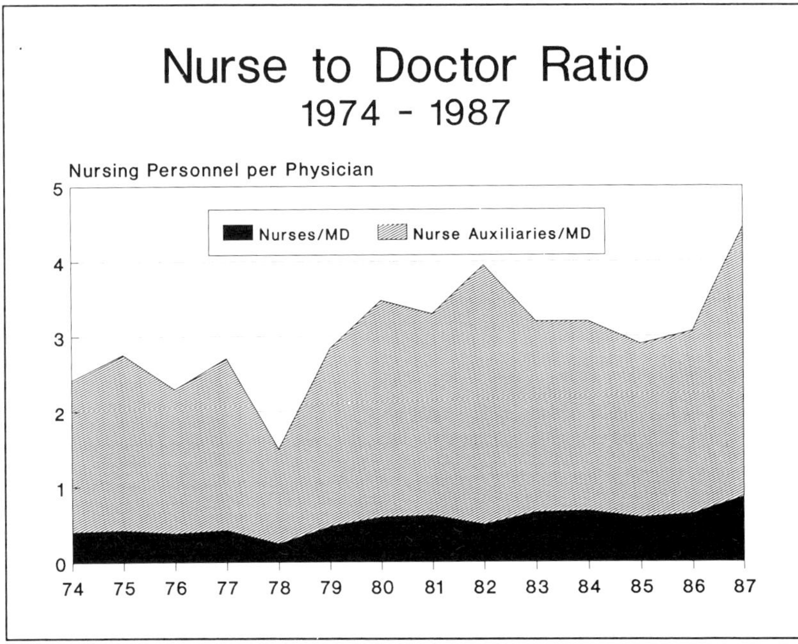

Despite a plan to increase the nurse-to-doctor ratio, there is still fewer than one nurse and only three auxiliary nurses for each physician.

1976 Nicaragua had 39 professional nurses per 100 doctors; by 1984 this had improved to 55 per hundred, but still lagged behind the rate for Central America of 68 per hundred (see Figure 10.3). In industrialised countries, by contrast, nurses almost invariably outnumber doctors: in the United States, for example, there are four professional nurses for every doctor.

The shortage of nurses is acutely felt in primary health care, but it is even more serious in hospitals. In 1985, 43% of the nurses needed in primary care were available, compared with only 31% in hospitals.[23] The number of nurses and nursing auxiliaries has failed to keep pace with the increase in hospital beds. Between 1980 and 1983, the number of hospital beds increased by 546, but the number of nurses working in hospitals by only 171, and the number of auxiliaries by 176. The shortage is greatest in the five new hospitals opened since 1979. Some of these institutions have been so short of nursing staff that the opening of new wards has been delayed for months or years. The shortage of nurses, especially in hospitals, is due in part to MINSA's policy of investing heavily in the training of large numbers of doctors. Ironically, it is the doctors themselves, who realise that hospital-based medicine depends largely on nursing staff, who are now demanding improved conditions for nurses.

Many of the problems facing nurses in Nicaragua are similar to those found in industrialised countries. Nursing is a relatively neglected profession. Salaries are poor, training facilities are inadequate, training is frequently isolated from practice, and working conditions are often extremely difficult. Poor promotion opportunities in the nursing system makes medicine relatively more attractive for rapid advancement. Despite heavy competition for entrance to medical school, nursing school classes have been undersubscribed since 1984. The profession has failed to attract many male trainees.

The poor quality of working relations with doctors further discourages people from becoming nurses. Many doctors assume that nurses know little and so pay little attention to their views. It is common for doctors not to explain to nurses the medical orders they have written. When challenged on their diagnosis or treatment, obscure claims of 'medical criteria' discourage nurses and give them little motivation to collaborate closely with doctors. Former Health Minister Lea Guido made efforts to change this situation by leading an educational effort to develop teamwork and 'treat each patient like your own mother or father'. But the heart of the problem was the quality of relations between doctors and nurses, which is changing only slowly.

Unlike the doctors, nurses have not been able to exert much influence on the political process. The weakness of organised nursing was seen in the closure of the university level nursing programme in 1983, the elimination of the national nursing office in the Ministry of Health in 1985, and the lowering of training qualification requirements in 1986.[24] Vehement opposition to these moves by the nurses' professional association *El Colegio de Enfermeras* led to the establishment of a national advisory group on nursing in 1988.[25] This group has succeeded in re-establishing the three-year basic programme for nursing education, expanding the training options available, increasing some salary levels, and allowing nurses to enter a post-graduate programme in epidemiology.

MINSA policy is now to employ two nurses and three auxiliaries for each doctor. To meet this goal, nurses are now being trained at six regional hospitals and auxiliaries are trained in one-year programmes in each region of the country.[26] Even so, undersubscribed classes and rapid abandonment of the nursing field will delay the improvement in the doctor-nurse ratio for at least a decade.

New priorities

In 1987 there were 1,955 physicians in Nicaragua. They included 300 general practitioners, 637 specialists (including 103 from other countries), 283 interns, 280 residents, and 455 carrying out their two-year social service requirement. About 1,300 doctors, 1,300 professional nurses, and

3,800 nursing auxiliaries had been trained since 1979.

A rapid increase in the numbers of doctors trained was a political necessity in the first years of the revolution. It was a long-held dream of social reformers and responded to the felt needs of both organised medicine and the population as a whole. It also enabled MINSA to cope with the emigration of almost half the doctors working in Nicaragua before 1979. But does it make sense for Nicaragua to continue to train so many new doctors? While the country can certainly use them, their training is many times more costly than that of paramedical personncl. A large group of paramedical personnel could be trained more rapidly, would cost less to employ, and would probably be more willing to live and work in isolated rural communities, outlying regions and poor neighbourhoods.

Given the relatively small number of students qualified to enter university, it is also questionable whether admitting 500 students every year into medicine is the most effective use of scarce human resources. These students might well serve the country more effectively in fields such as engineering, agriculture, or public administration. And although newly graduated doctors may be able to bring health care to people who have never had any before, they also generate more demand for expensive medicines and supplies.[27] With these concerns in mind, MINSA in 1989 began to restrict the size of new medical school classes to 150 per year.

Despite MINSA's best efforts to retain the country's doctors, at least half of those trained before 1979 have left the country during the past decade. Most have found work in the United States, Mexico, Panama and Venezuela. Some, however, miss the status and respect they enjoyed in Nicaragua and return to their old posts after some months abroad.

If there were no shortage of doctors, the political pressure they exert might be less. Most worrying is the emigration of specialists trained since 1979. An end to the war and an upturn in the economy would make the prospect of staying in the country more attractive. In the meantime, however, the Government is obliged to reduce the number of specialists being trained and apply stricter criteria for the selection of candidates. At the same time, it will continue to pay increased attention to the interests of doctors, and will attempt to improve further their already privileged social and political status.

Chapter 11: Medicines and Medical Equipment

"MINSA announces that, beginning on 15 March, there will be a charge for medicines that are dispensed at health centres throughout the country. With this measure, MINSA hopes to control the indiscriminate use of medicines."
(From Radio Sandino broadcast, 7 March 1986.)

Under the Somozas, the provision of pharmaceuticals was left to the invisible hand of the free market. Predictably, the Somoza family was heavily involved in that market through ownership of SOLKA, the country's second largest pharmaceutical company. Drugs were promoted like cigarettes or Coca Cola through advertisements on billboards and radio, and in newspapers and magazines. Doctors and pharmacists earned special premiums for promoting the products of particular drug companies. In addition, the political domination of the US-allied elite created a strong image of the American 'good life' which dominated the media and popular culture. The result was what is now referred to as the 'culture of medicines'. In the minds of the general public and medical leaders, the more drugs they took and the higher the doses used, the better. This commercialism had reached absurd proportions. A popular B vitamin complex, Neurobion, sold for 38 *cordobas* a vial, while an identical formula marketed under the name Vitalgia sold for 14 *cordobas* but was much less popular. Almost no-one taking either formula could derive any possible health benefit from it.

But there was also another side to the story. While affluent Nicaraguans and Social Security beneficiaries consumed too many drugs, most other people remained largely dependent on home remedies and traditional medicines using plants, roots, powders and the secret potions of folk healers. Especially in rural areas, there was almost no access to modern drugs.

With the advent of the revolution, everyone wanted to fill their medicine cabinets. Doctors often responded by providing unnecessary injections and drugs on demand for simple ailments that required little or no medication at all. For a child with influenza, for example, doctors commonly prescribed two antibiotics, an analgesic, multivitamins and a tonic. None of this was needed and much of it was harmful. The revolution's health system had to respond to the people's felt needs, but at what cost? If the people wanted too many expensive, ineffective, or dangerous medicines, should the government provide them? Breaking the grip of the 'drug mentality' would prove to be a singularly daunting task.

Free drugs for all?

In July 1979, within days of taking power, the new Government decreed that all drugs dispensed in public hospitals and health centres would be free of charge. More than any other act, this decree convinced the population that the health services were theirs. The full financial implications of this policy were not yet clear, however, and the Government soon found itself retreating from it bit by bit.

The top priority was to provide essential drugs to those who previously had little or no access to them. The rapid expansion of the primary care system between 1979 and 1983 (see Chapter 3), especially in rural areas, meant that essential drugs could be provided by pharmacies in hospitals and health centres. As MINSA concentrated on opening new health centres and getting doctors and nurses to staff them, lack of organisation was the rule in the pharmaceutical system. Millions of dollars' worth of drugs were imported on credit. Many of these medicines as well as products from the country's 20 private drug firms and countless petty importers and middle men found their way onto the black market. It was not unusual to see a private pharmacy run by a conservative opponent of the Sandinistas whose shelves were stocked with donated Cuban products.

Although supplying the rural areas was sometimes a problem, the real nightmare was in the cities. Queues outside hospital pharmacies backed out into the streets. Doctors filled a sheet full of prescriptions, only about 60% of which could be found in any given hospital, and patients began to migrate from one hospital to another in search of all the drugs they were prescribed. This meant that the public health system, above all the hospitals, was distributing so many medicines that supplies were usually short.

Middle-class patients complained most vigorously about empty pharmacy shelves. The case of Byron Molina, the wealthiest landowner in Jinotega, was typical. He visited a foreign doctor at the local health centre complaining of indigestion and asking for an American antacid, Mylanta. Since this brand was not available the doctor wrote a prescription for aluminium and magnesium hydroxide, the generic name for the same product. He flatly refused to accept the prescription. Since the medicine was from Cuba he presumed it to be poor quality and waited until relatives sent him the medicine from the US.

Fig. 11.1

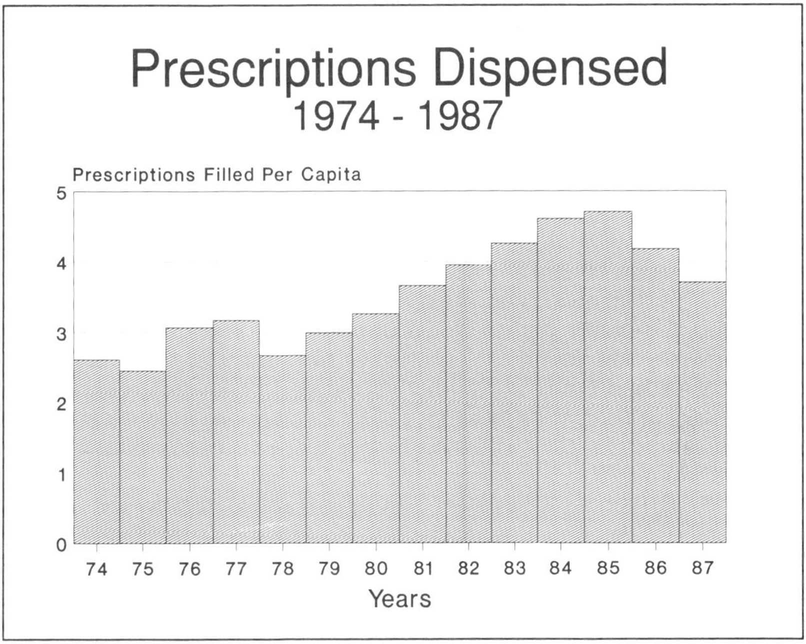

The number of prescriptions dispensed per capita nearly doubled between the 1970s and the 1980s.

From 1980 to 1982, private pharmacies increased their share of the burgeoning drug market from 59% to 85%. To decongest hospital pharmacies and to provide a source of over-the-counter medicines for the urban poor, 30 public pharmacies were opened in 1983 and 31 more in the next five years. About 60% of the people surveyed in and around Managua in 1984 said that they obtained medicines from either these pharmacies or primary care facilities,[1] because supply was similar to the private pharmacies but prices were subsidised. Another 20% reported buying medicines on the open market, while a similar proportion reported buying from *curanderos* (folk healers).

In a somewhat chaotic fashion, basic drugs (as well as other medicines) became much more widely available after 1979. In 1981, for example, more than 10 million prescriptions were dispensed, representing a near doubling from the yearly average before 1978.[2] The number of prescriptions peaked in 1985 at more than 15 million (see Figure 11.1). Yet demand was rising even faster than supply, and widespread complaints were heard about the growing unavailability of medicines.

Despite excessive use of medicines, the reduced prices and wide availability of pharmaceuticals since 1979 have helped many. This is most apparent in rural areas. Bosco Liviana is a peasant farmer in Matagalpa. In 1985 he started becoming thin, weak and had a persistent cough. He did not need a doctor to tell him what was happening — he had tuberculosis. He knew this because his father and brother had died from tuberculosis in the 1970s when they could only occasionally afford to purchase the antibiotics to treat it. (Interruptions in treatment promote resistant strains of the tubercular bacillus such as the one which Bosco contracted.) He started to visit a health post as he could get a fairly steady supply of appropriate antibiotics there at no cost. Buying these from a pharmacy would have taken most of his annual income. He has had no symptoms since 1987 and is now considered cured.[3]

Public pharmacies even took turns providing a 24-hour service, something the health centres would offer only four years later. Yet the Government soon found that providing free drugs sapped the health system of needed funds and further encouraged the overconsumption of unnecessary or dangerous medicines. The value of one month's imported pharmaceuticals in 1982 equalled that of a whole year's drug imports during the late 1970s.

In March 1982 the Ministry of Health imposed a 'registration fee' for prescriptions; the drugs themselves were still free. In 1986, a more radical shift occurred: there would be a charge for prescription medicines, albeit heavily subsidised. Not all drugs would be charged for, however. Those needed in special programmes, such as tuberculosis, venereal disease control and immunisation, would still be free, as would drugs for hospital in-patients.

As a result, some people stopped visiting the clinics and health centres; any prescription fee was prohibitive for them. Yet the new policy still left a huge gap between drugs sold at 'official' prices through government health facilities and drugs sold 'commercially' by private pharmacies. Between March 1982 and June 1987, for example, the cost to patients of essential drugs sold at government health facilities was only about 25% of their commercial value. This glaring discrepancy led to two serious problems.

First, some popular drugs sold out rapidly each month and for weeks at a time there were none to be bought. Hospitals and health centres had an average of only 60% to 70% of all programmed medicines in stock.[4] Second, 'professional' patients were able to make a living by obtaining drugs at official rates and then selling them on the black market for much higher prices. In a campaign called the 'war against the ants', health leaders tried to identify and educate those who abused the health system in this way.[5] It turned out that many of the culprits were health workers who were labelled 'white coat bandits'.

Subsidised prices stimulated many forms of black market activity. Near the northern and southern borders, people opened lively resale trades with Honduran and Costa Rican traders. The most 'black marketed' drugs were contraceptives. Since supply from government sources was irregular, doctors providing family planning services in clinics around the country sometimes had to go to the open-air markets in Managua and buy pills on the black market, in order to provide them to clinic patients.[6] The pills were usually purchased at public pharmacies in the first place, and sold to traders in the market.

To deal with these inter-related problems, the Government resorted to a measure which, only a few years earlier, would have been regarded as political heresy. In 1987 subsidies were slashed to abolish the difference between essential drugs sold through official and commercial channels. Essential drugs, however, still received an indirect subsidy through the variable exchange rate system. The elimination of direct subsidies meant that except for several special disease control programmes, the prices of essential drugs at government health facilities and private pharmacies were generally the same. Private pharmacies continued to sell more non-essential, or 'popular' drugs, which provided them with the bulk of their profits.

The policy took another turn when a single rate of exchange was established in the national monetary reform of February 1988. Intended as an emergency measure to attack inflation and improve the business environment, it also eliminated the indirect subsidy for medicines. The effect was a five-fold increase in the price paid by the consumer. The public's reaction was immediate. After ever-rising consumption of medicines for the previous nine years, the sales of medicines plummeted. "There is a drastic reduction in demand", said Byron Ramirez of the Ministry of Internal Commerce. "If someone needs ten pills, at best he'll only be able to buy five now." Medicine sales fell so drastically that prices had to be cut by 35 - 50% to avoid the products becoming outdated prior to sale.

The high cost of drugs

Nicaragua's drug bill is much too high. The per capita annual cost of medicines in Nicaragua is about $20. In the years 1980 to 1983, pharmaceutical imports averaged $50 million a year. If the rate of growth seen in these years had continued, it would have led to a drug import bill of $100 million a year by 1990.[7] In 1985, Nicaragua spent $31 million on importing drugs or the products to manufacture them. This was equivalent to the value of the country's cotton crop (its second biggest export).

The reasons for excessive costs were identified as early as 1981.[8] First, over 90% of all products used to make finished medicines are imported. At least 80% come only from capitalist countries, where the terms of trade for developing countries are unfavourable. Nicaragua routinely pays two to five times more for its drug imports than necessary.

In 1986 the Pan American Health Organisation (PAHO) established a programme to enable all Central American countries to purchase essential drugs in bulk at competitive prices on the world market.[9] With a grant of $4 million from the Dutch Government, PAHO set up FORMED — a revolving loan fund through which each country can obtain 16 essential drugs, to a total value of $650,000. PAHO procures the drugs in bulk, paying only one-quarter to one-third of the average price normally paid by the Central American Governments. The Governments then reimburse PAHO, making two rounds of bulk purchases annually.

Essential drugs

Reducing the vast number of medicines on sale could save at least $5 million a year. In the late 1970s about 3,500 pharmaceutical products were registered and available. These included, for example, 52 different types of ampicillin preparations. Many unregistered products — the so-called 'popular' drugs — were also readily available. Apart from narcotics, any drug could be purchased without a doctor's prescription. There was some logic in this, since most of the people never saw a doctor. But with a multiplicity of drugs on sale in shops, supermarkets, market stalls and pharmacies, the inevitable result was widespread self-medication using drugs that were either useless (such as Vitamin B12 injections) or harmful (such as chloramphenicol).

In 1977 an Expert Committee of the World Health Organisation published a *Model List of Essential Drugs* which recommended 220 drugs and vaccines as essential in good medical practice. All were of proven safety and efficacy and possessed well-understood therapeutic properties. Most were no longer protected by patent and could be produced in large quantities at reasonable cost. It seemed logical for Nicaragua to develop its own list of essential drugs, based on the WHO model list, taking into account local epidemiological, pharmacological and economic factors.

In 1981 the Ministry of Health began to develop its own list of essential drugs. The project met with immediate hostility from many doctors, who saw the list as a threat to their freedom to prescribe. Domestic and foreign pharmaceutical companies feared for their profits. Even patients were mobilised to resist the plan. Many people relied on a trusted brand name; consumers at all levels were encouraged to accept no substitutes for their tried and true product. Only in rural areas, where preferences for particular brand names had not yet developed, were Cuban and eastern European pharmaceutical products readily accepted.

Finally, after widespread and painstaking consultations, a National Pharmaceutical Formulary was published with 667 products in 1984.[10] It designated the number and types of drugs to be supplied at each level of the health system, based on the training of health workers at that level. In 1985 the Formulary was reduced to 475 products, of which only 65 were listed as indispensable for general use. Another 343 were reserved for specialists with access to diagnostic facilities, and a further 76 were designated as 'high risk' drugs to be used only under strict protocols. In 1988 a revised Formulary was prepared, consisting of 392 products, of which 253 items were designated for distribution only by prescription.

At each step, organised medicine opposed the implementation of the various formularies. As a result, the lists have been observed mainly in the breach. Private importers continue to import and sell any medicine without official sanction. At the end of 1988, for example, both public and private pharmacies had ample supplies of useless products such as injectable Vitamin B12. At the same time, pharmacies ran out of birth control pills and were unable to obtain further supplies. The formulary has, however, had some impact on the urban and rural health posts, where at least half of the 65 'indispensable' medicines are usually available.

Local production and distribution

Increased local drug production could reduce the drug bill even though production costs are high because of Nicaragua's limited domestic market and lack of export opportunities, reducing the potential for economies of scale. Heavy investment in technically sophisticated equipment is also needed to ensure good quality control. The promotion of self-reliance in medicines would create employment, help to establish an industrial base, and reduce dependence on unpredictable outside markets. Reducing the percentage of medicines which are imported as finished products to 40% would reduce costs by about $5 million a year.

In 1984 COFARMA was formed to manage the importation and distribution of all drugs and raw materials for local production. COFARMA supplies 14 privately-owned drug manufacturers and two state-owned firms: SOLKA and Laboratorios Populares. Since the trade embargo imposed by the US in May 1985, Nicaragua has imported raw materials for its pharmaceutical industry mainly from Spain, Holland, socialist countries and Mexico.

Local drug production is concentrated on 100 of the products listed in Nicaragua's National Formulary of Essential Drugs. SOLKA produces only essential drugs; the private companies produce non-essential, or 'popular', drugs as well. More than 60% of all medicines consumed are still imported as finished products.[11]

SOLKA receives foreign aid in the form of equipment, technical expertise, money and basic materials from countries such as Holland, Argentina, Italy and Spain. Nevertheless, SOLKA works at only 40% of its potential capacity and has never provided more than 20% of the country's essential drug needs. There are continuous shortages of basic materials and spare parts to repair old machinery. In addition, low salaries make it difficult to recruit the highly specialised staff needed to manage a drug company. While private drug firms can offer higher salaries, they also suffer from a lack of basic materials and spare parts, and their production levels are well below their capacity.

Although state-controlled, COFARMA has considerable independence and pays salaries comparable to those in the private sector. COFARMA distributes about 80% of the drugs imported to government health facilities and 20% to private pharmacies. All drugs — whether purchased or donated — are first stored in Managua and then distributed to stores in each of the regions. COFARMA's warehouse, bookkeeping, and inventory practices have put an end to large-scale medicine thefts. Production and distribution, however, still lack the efficiency needed. Vice-Minister of Health Pablo Coca observed in 1987 that 2.5% of funds for medicines were wasted by deterioration, lack of attention to the expiry dates, or theft. About $3 million could be saved from improved administrative efficiency. According to Byron Ramirez, "Sometimes emergency importation is necessary, such as when dengue fever broke out in 1986. Medicines were bought quickly on the open market, in dollars. By the time our factories could produce the required medicines, the market was already flooded with imports."

Local supply, particularly in war zones and other rural areas, is also a problem. On 14 July 1988, for example, *Contras* attacked a convoy of trucks carrying medicines and other supplies to the small town of Mancotal, near the Honduras border. No-one, including the local priest, risked a resupply operation for fear of another attack. It was two months before a *brigadista* from a neighbouring area was persuaded to take on the task.

Overconsumption

Despite improved coordination of distribution and the elimination of subsidised prices, Nicaraguans still often consume medicines which are ineffective or harmful. Antibiotics make up 60% of imported medicines. Enough antibiotics are consumed to provide each person with five full courses of treatment a year — more than is used by people in Europe or the US. But people often take antibiotics for only one or two days at a time, making each dose ineffective and promoting resistant bacterial strains. With the recent elimination of pharmaceutical subsidies, the tendency to take less than a full course of treatment is even greater.

Part of the problem of over-consumption has been the easy availability of a wide variety of drugs on the open market. It was not until June 1987 that the Government issued a regulation making a doctor's prescription necessary for all essential drugs, including those sold by private pharmacies. The large private sector and black market in medicines make it difficult to ensure enforcement of this regulation. The Government still has no control over non-essential drugs, which remain on the open market. In February 1988 a researcher from the Central American University in Managua found a wide range of potentially dangerous drugs on sale:[12]

"In supermarkets aspirin, high-powered antibiotics and all kinds of other medicines have been sold — and are still being sold — on the same shelves as buttons and crackers. Ampicillin and Vitamin B complex are everyone's favourite self-prescribed medicines for whatever disorder, no matter how light or serious. For mental exhaustion or migraine, Vitamin B injections; for indigestion however caused, Milk of Magnesia; for any degree of flu, ampicillin by the dozens and for nervous tension, Valium."

The 'drug mentality' affects both doctors and the public. In a 1984 survey, more than half of those responding believed that coloured pills were more effective than white pills. The pressure on medical practitioners to over-prescribe drugs is intense: a doctor who advises bed rest and plenty of fluids instead of prescribing several drugs for a common cold may be called a 'quack'. Worse, patients may believe that he or she is against the revolution in denying them what are believed to be essential health services.

Efforts to improve doctors' prescribing habits have had only limited success. Most doctors receive little training in pharmacology and are unprepared to make optimal choices. Large numbers of patients and poor diagnostic capacities leave over-prescribing the most expedient solution for a harried clinician. This also avoids confrontations with patients, many of whom are convinced of the need for a particular injection and are unwilling to accept 'no' for an answer.

At the pharmacy of the Granada hospital, staff are now protected from

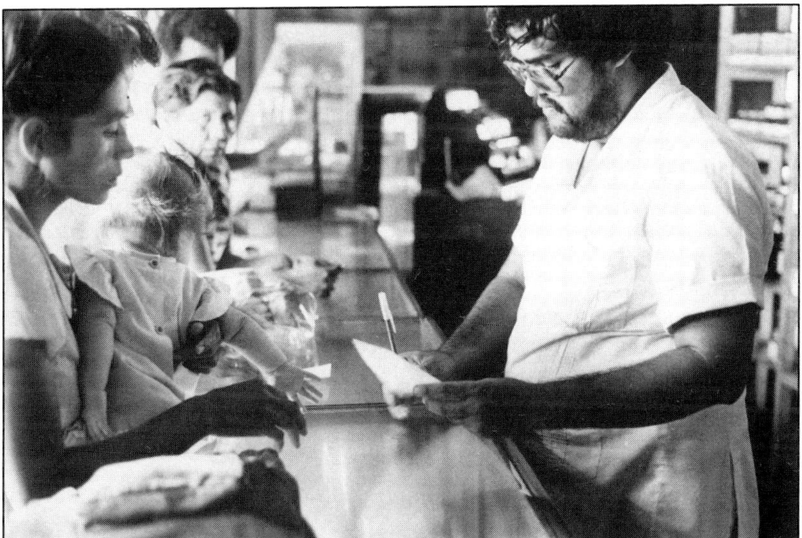

GLEN WILLIAMS

Many Nicaraguans still suffer from a 'drug mentality' which creates unnecessary demands on the health services. Pharmacists are often at the receiving end of complaints from patients when drugs are unavailable.

the public by an iron grille. "The people receive medicines prepacked and complain that they don't get enough. They shout at the girls," according to pharmacy director Fidelia Arguello. "Not long ago one of the patients beat up one of our pharmacy staff — that's how agitated they get." One specialist invariably prescribes 84 capsules of Ampicillin. The hospital pharmacy, however, follows a policy of giving only 16 capsules at a time to avoid over-prescribing. "This leads to conflicts with both patients and doctors. Every month we discuss with the hospital staff the problems of drugs and prescriptions, but they don't listen. On the other hand, patients are seldom satisfied either."

Traditional medicine

The Health Minister suggests that one solution to the problem of the over-consumption of drugs is to "replace the culture of antibiotics with our older culture of herbs. We need to remember camomile, bitter orange, savila, and pasote." Traditional health care in Nicaragua is not as well-developed as it is in countries such as Guatemala, where the large indigenous population has maintained a long pharmaceutical tradition. Since 1986 health educators have led an effort to recover and systematise information on herbal medicines in rural Nicaragua. Much of this knowledge resides with traditional birth attendants and has only recently been researched systematically.

There are many views on the value of traditional medicine. Decentralisation, the economic crisis, and an inability to meet the demand for modern medicines have encouraged experimentation in this area. In 1985 a botanical pharmacy was started in Esteli. Among its activities was a national meeting in which more than 900 school students and teachers presented the results of 3,000 interviews with people about herbal medicine.[13] The pharmacy has also drawn up an inventory of herbal resources and has classified 325 medicinal plants. These, in turn, are being tested in biochemistry laboratories in Europe. A cooperative farm outside Esteli grows, packages, and sells about a dozen of the most popular herbal remedies.

In August 1987 the Ministers of Health of the seven Central American countries, meeting in Managua, issued a declaration stating that the time was ripe for the integration of traditional and local health systems. In November 1987 the first Central American meeting for the 'rescue of traditional medicine' was held in Esteli.[14] These initiatives, together with the formal training of traditional *parteras* (see Chapter 8), reflect increased official awareness of the potential contribution of traditional medicine to health. "We don't want to overdo it. We can't try to use these medications to treat every kind of pathology or illness", says Health Minister Dora Maria Tellez. "But we've had good results. Once the study is finished and the war is over, we plan ... to cultivate more of these plants commercially."

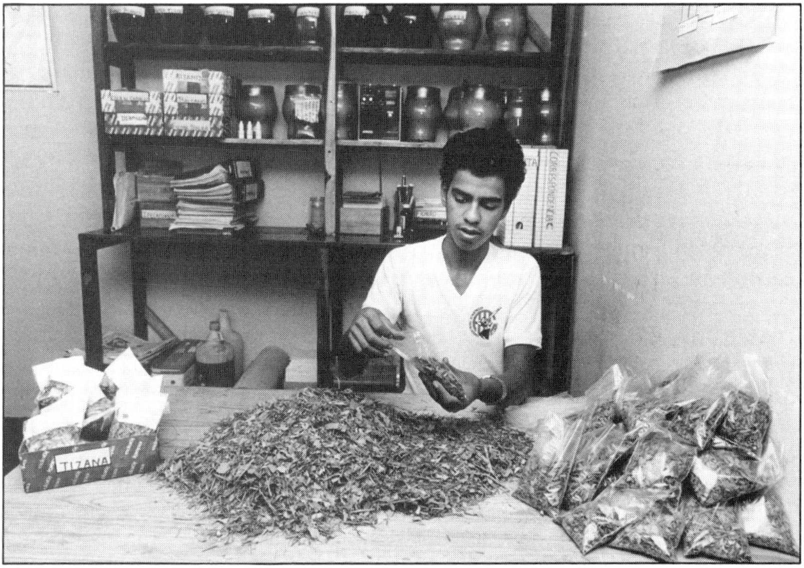

ANA CECILIA GONZALES

Packing medicinal herbs for traditional remedies in the pharmacy at Esteli. Research into the effectiveness of herbal medicines is being undertaken and their increasing use could help cut the drug import bill.

Equipment and supplies

Laboratory equipment is an essential component of modern health care.[15] In hospitals and clinics, over 1,000 products are used in diagnosis and treatment. Unlike pharmaceuticals, most of these can be purchased locally. Given the strong public demand for medicines, however, this area has received less priority. While 90% of the drug purchases planned for 1987 were made, only 60% of materials (such as sheets, bandages and cleaning supplies), 50% of lab reagents, and 60% of the small instruments in the plan were purchased.[16]

For months at a time none of the five blood-gas machines in Managua works. The only way to get an indication of the oxygen perfusion of the blood at such times is to look at it in a syringe to judge its brightness. The haemodialysis unit in Managua has been out of commission most of the time since 1980 for lack of parts. Old X-ray machines produce pictures so dim as to be of questionable utility: twins have been delivered on several occasions following an X-ray which showed only one faint foetal skull. A similar situation is found with the one cobalt-based cancer treatment unit. A waiting list of six months for therapy is in effect, partly because the cobalt bomb is so old that patients must lie under it for an hour or more to receive an effective dose.

The most serious bottlenecks in the health system are caused by the slow repair of equipment.[17] This was a serious problem before the war; the severing of credit and commercial relations by the US has made the repair of most of the country's medical equipment even more difficult. It is estimated that 70% of the medical equipment in the country is from the US. Of the four hospitals in the north-central region of the country, sterilisers for surgical equipment are usually out of service in two. This results in delays in surgery, higher infection rates, and high transport costs in taking equipment from one hospital to another for sterilisation. Sometimes private trucks must be rented to transport resterilised surgical equipment. Laboratory equipment in health centres may take up to a year to repair.

In 1987 MINSA took its first complete inventory. It found that there were about 4,000 pieces of electronic equipment for direct patient care and diagnosis,[18] of which 20-30% were out of service at any given time. Hospitals and health centres depended on 257 pieces of electromechanical equipment, of which 40-50% were out of service.

The inventory also showed that MINSA ran 83 operating rooms of which 12 were out of service, 63 X-ray machines of which more than a third were not functioning, and 112 clinical laboratories, most of which had some non-functioning equipment.

The training and social service practice of local doctors prepares them for some of these limitations. Dr. Rodolfo Correa is doing his social service at the health centre in Matiguas, Matagalpa:

"A Nicaraguan doctor is a clinical doctor. To diagnose amoebiasis, we don't need a test. We check to see if the stool has some mucus, is bloody, watery, green, or yellow...To diagnose diabetes, we will ask a patient, 'How have you been feeling? Are you thirsty?' It's guerrilla medicine. We sometimes make mistakes, and sometimes we do well. Everything is a fight. We improvise."

Transportation is more problematic. In 1987 MINSA owned 87 ambulances, 369 pickup trucks and jeeps, 63 large trucks, 26 vans, 12 small buses, 38 cars, four trailer trucks, one tractor, five river boats, 22 motor boats, and 23 bicycles. About 35% of these vehicles were out of service at any given time. Repair is made more difficult by the wide variety of donations and purchases received. MINSA's vehicles come from 28 manufacturers and include 188 different models. Poor skill among drivers is another problem. In 1986, MINSA vehicles were involved in 114 accidents.

Balancing priorities

Misuse and over-consumption of medicines weaken the health system and use up funds which are needed to repair and maintain transportation, supplies, and essential medicines. Elimination of misuse and over-consumption of medicines will, however, require a great deal of education. Both health professionals and consumers will need to understand better the uses and limitations of antibiotics, pain relievers, and vitamins. This will require cultural and technical education over an extended period of time.

Despite the serious misuse and high cost of medicines, Nicaragua remains one of the few Latin American countries where essential pharmaceuticals are available most of the time at urban and rural primary care facilities. The massive effort and repeated organisational and administrative changes made to keep the medicines flowing is an expression of the Government's high commitment to meeting such basic needs.

Chapter 12: Financing Health

"The truth is that we have never had the financial capacity to meet our needs. International assistance will continue to be needed for the foreseeable future. But it is up to us to determine the priorities."
(Vice-Minister of Health, Dr. Milton Valdez)

Health systems in developing countries are difficult to scrutinise with economic analysis.[1] Key information is often unavailable, and few health leaders have a complete overview of monetary issues. Despite such shortcomings, it is possible to trace the development of health finance in Nicaragua from the early days of relative affluence in the early 1980s to the present state of financial crisis.

How much should health care cost?
This question confronted MINSA when a budget was to be developed for 1980. Since no reliable data on the Somoza period were available, officials guessed at the budget of the pre-revolutionary agencies dealing with health and then doubled that amount. Compared with most other developing countries, Nicaragua was already investing heavily in health prior to the revolution. During most of the 1970s the health sector absorbed about 8% of the Government's budget (see Figure 12.1). This was double the average level of health budgets in developing countries. The health sector represented 1-2% of the national Gross Domestic Product (GDP), a higher proportion than in any other Central American country except Costa Rica.

With the revolution, health investment rose rapidly. By 1981 the health sector represented 13% of the Government's budget and 4.7% of the GDP. Despite rising inflation, the value of public funds invested in health also rose rapidly.

After 1984, further increases in the number of *cordobas* devoted to the health system were eaten up by inflation. By 1986 MINSA had only slightly more inflation-adjusted *cordobas* to spend than it did in 1980.

Fig. 12.1

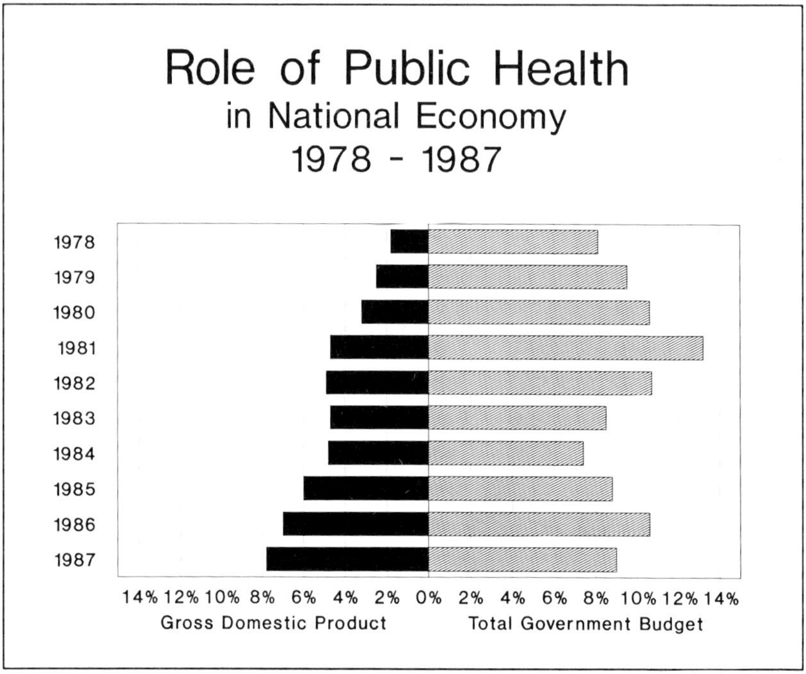

The Health Ministry has taken a large share of the Government's budget since the late 1970s. As the budget represented an increasing proportion of the country's economy in the 1980s, the proportional role of health in the national economy has similarly grown.

Yet compared to the other Central American countries, including Costa Rica where economic problems have been less severe, the Nicaraguan health sector has fared very well. In the other countries of the region, health funding was severely cut back in the 1980s (see Figure 12.2).

Budgetary changes

Despite rising military spending throughout the 1980s, the health sector maintained its prominent position in the national budget. In 1982, 19% of public expenditure went to the military (see Figure 12.3). This rose to 46% of the budget in 1987. Despite a serious reduction in availability of funds to other sectors, the social sector in general, and the health sector in particular, were largely spared from cuts prior to 1988. "It may seem contradictory", said a government planner, "that although the war costs us more, we need to invest in the health system to reduce the war's impact on the general population." Maintaining a high level of investment in health, in the context of a shrinking national economy, increased

Fig. 12.2

Economic Recession
and Changes in Health Spending

Country:	Per Capita GDP (1980 - 1984)	Per Capita Health Spending (1980 - 1985)
Guatemala	-15%	-58%
El Salvador	-26%	-32%
Costa Rica	-12%	-17%
Honduras	-12%	-15%
Nicaragua*	-65%	- 2%

*Calculated with offical inflation index

Sources: Direccion de Finanza, MINSA. Ministerio de Finanza, JGN. Cornia GA, Jolly R, Stewart F, *Adjustment with a human face*, Oxford: Clarendon, 1987.

MINSA's relative share of the Gross Domestic Product from 1-1.5% in the 1970s to 7.8% in 1987 (see Figure 12.1).

Sources of domestic funds

Prior to the revolution, the largest pool of health funds was generated by the social security system (see Figure 12.4). Since 1979 these payroll deductions have continued to fund health services, which are now open to the whole population. A unique arrangement was made to transfer 9% of all social security deductions to MINSA for its general operating budget in what came to be known as the 'solidarity fund'. Social security health funds in 1978 represented 65% of all health expenditure. Increasing investments from other sources reduced the relative value of this pool to 30% of MINSA's budget in 1980, 28% in 1983, and 19% in 1986.

National lotteries are also used to fund health systems in many Latin American countries.[2] In Nicaragua it is estimated that 3-4% of the health budget is provided by funds generated by the lottery. Domestic charitable donations were an important informal source of operating funds prior to the revolution, possibly amounting to as much as 10% of the budget, but the size and variety of programmes since 1979 have dwarfed this source.

International funds were an important source of income in the early 1980s, particularly an Interamerican Development Bank loan to construct

Fig. 12.3

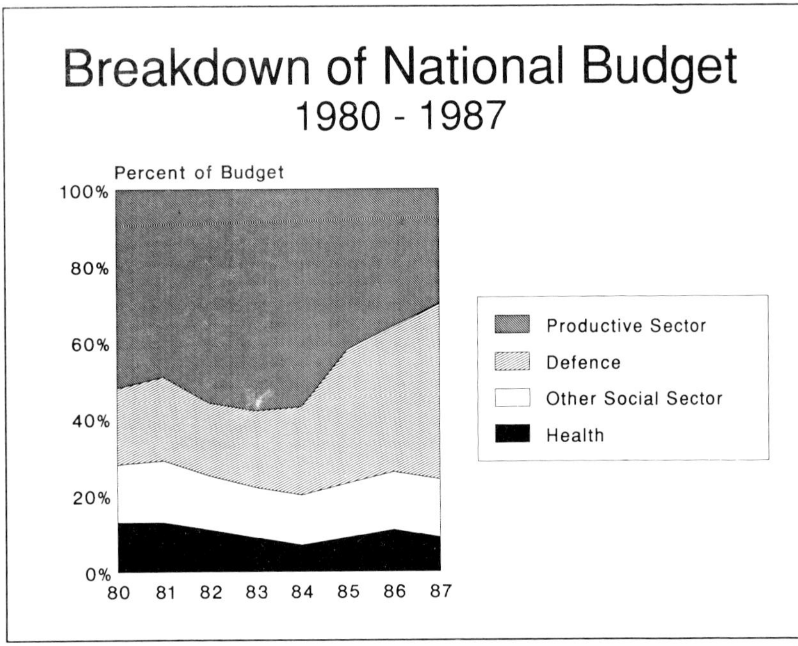

Health and other social sector spending were largely spared, although defence took an increasing proportion of the national budget in the late 1980s.

health facilities. Such funds made up 20% of MINSA's budget in 1981, but diminished to 6% in 1984. US Government efforts to block any further grants or loans have been largely successful: direct dollar donations for health have been a minor portion of MINSA's budget since 1985.

A decrease in the value of international loans, domestic charity and social security funds has left central government to provide an increasing proportion of the health sector budget. In 1987 the Government provided about 80% of all funds for the MINSA budget. Even after being cut by 30% in January 1989, health continued to receive more than 10% of the total government budget. Such high dependence on regular government funds highlights the importance of the Government's commitment to health.[3]

Destination of health funds

The apportionment of the health budget has changed little since 1980. The largest single component has always been the hospitals, taking up about half the entire budget. On average, each of the 31 hospitals utilises

Fig. 12.4

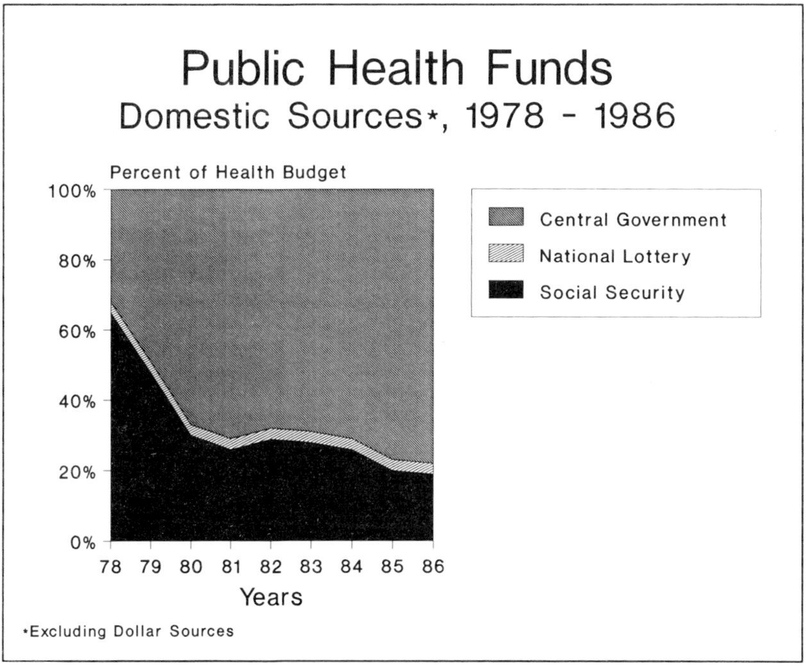

Central government provided an increasing proportion of all funds for the health sector as the value of social security contributions declined.

1.5% of the national health budget. In 1983 MINSA began to shift funds toward primary care. This trend slowed in 1984 when falling quality of care in hospitals, in addition to war-related demands, dictated a return to traditional funding patterns. Nonetheless, funding for primary health care showed an overall expansion from 14% in 1981 to 26% in 1987.

The main victim of the health budget cut in the late 1980s was administration. Decentralisation had already helped to reduce the cost of administration from 25% in 1981 to 14% in 1986. Preventive components of the MINSA budget receive smaller funding allotments. Health education and malaria control together account for about 8% of the total budget. International funding of the health budget has been concentrated on these latter components and on primary health care.

Nearly half of all *cordoba* funds are destined for salaries. Most of the rest goes for equipment and supplies. Because of the preferential rates of exchange applied through 1988 and the availability of donations to reduce overall costs, medicines distributed by the health system appeared to cost relatively little. Their *cordoba* value was only about as much as food consumed by patients and less than other medical supplies. Investments in construction and repair of facilities consume the rest of the budget. Expenditure on construction peaked at 14% of the budget in 1982 and declined to 1% in 1986.

Imports

The economic crisis is reflected in a scarcity of dollars and imported goods. Health, more than other social sectors, depends on imported goods such as pharmaceuticals, spare parts and equipment, books and journals, reagents, expert consultations, and medical care for patients requiring treatment outside the country.

By far the largest import purchase is pharmaceuticals. More than half of MINSA's $40-$60 million import bill each year is destined for medicines. In 1986, $18 million was spent on finished medical products and $12 million went on ingredients for medicines which would be finished in Nicaraguan processing plants. By contrast, $800,000 was used to purchase equipment, and $300,000 to purchase vehicles. A total of $3 million was used to purchase powdered milk, some of which was for use by MINSA, who could have done more to reduce popular demand for this commodity. Such imports took up resources which were needed elsewhere; for example it was estimated that $1.5 million would have been sufficient to repair most of the broken medical equipment in the country.

International donations

While the country receives $100-$150 million in international aid each year, little of this is designated to supply dollars for imports. Official, registered donations, totalling about $10 - $15 million, probably cover less than half of all imports for health. Donations of goods-in-kind considerably exceed donated currency. In 1986 MINSA programmes received $10 million in cash donations while UN-related organisations provided $13.5 million worth of health assistance,[4] Western European countries gave about $1 million in the form of medical aid, and medical solidarity groups in North America and Europe provided goods and other assistance to the value of about $3 million. Some 40% of all materials donated to MINSA were unsolicited.[5]

Donations in kind via medical scholarships provided a further estimated $800,000 in value. Medical teams and supplies provided for foreign-run hospitals by the Soviet Union, the German Democratic Republic, and Cuba were estimated to be worth $2.5 million in 1986.

A shortage of dollars

As the national currency has weakened with rampant inflation, the relative value of imported goods has grown and the importance of donations has skyrocketed. In 1987 the value of donations exceeded the value of the total national health budget at both black market and parallel

Fig. 12.5

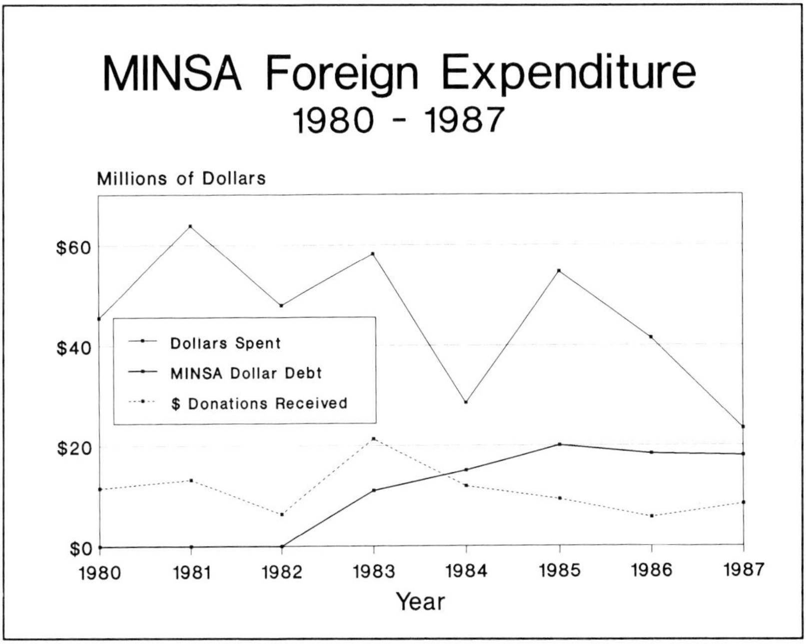

MINSA has spent considerably more US dollars for imports than it has received from international sources; thus, MINSA incurred a growing debt with the national Government during the mid-1980s.

market rates of exchange. Of course, the goods and services produced by the health system far exceed the real value of donations, but rampant inflation has made such comparisons meaningless. The economic embargo, the war and the declining economy have left the Government, and its health system, increasingly dependent on outside assistance.

The health system imports expensive goods for which it must pay in hard currency from central government funds. In 1987 more than two-thirds of all dollar purchases were paid for with central government funds. The commercial debt of MINSA begun in 1982 grew to about $20 million by 1987 (see Figure 12.5).

Reducing dollar dependence

Notable advances have been made by the health system in five areas to reduce the level of imports. First, an increasing proportion of medicines are being finished within the country: nearly all intravenous fluids, for example, are now fabricated nationally. Second, centralised purchasing and restriction in brands have helped rationalise supply. Together, these changes save the country about $5 million a year. Third, pesticide purchases have been reduced by more than half through revising the strategy for control of malaria, saving the country $1-$2 million a year. Fourth, innovations in the repair, re-use, or fabrication of spare parts save the country about $500,000 a year. Finally, the expanded use of herbal medicines makes an intangible but important contribution to reducing the demand for imported pharmaceuticals.

Value destroyed in the war

The health system has been hit hard by the *Contra* war. Great as the destruction has been, this represents only a small portion of the total destruction caused by the war. As in previous natural and man-made disasters in Nicaragua, most of the damage has been sustained by the agricultural and industrial sectors.

About 3% of all direct destruction in the *Contra* war was sustained by the health system. This includes $2 million for health posts and health centres, $2.8 million for ambulances and infrastructural facilities, and $1.2 million for medicines.[6]

While large stocks of medicines were destroyed in attacks on several health centres in 1984 and 1985, the greatest single loss occurred in the October 1983 bombing of the Pacific coast town of Corinto. In destroying the country's main oil depot, large warehouses with medicines, clothes, pesticides, and food worth several million dollars were lost.

MINSA estimated in January 1988 that reconstruction of destroyed facilities would cost 200 billion *cordobas*. This total was more than twice the current *cordoba* value of the country's annual health budget.

Put in the context of war-related destruction and the economic crisis gripping the country, the high commitment of the Sandinista Government to maintain its investment in health is all the more remarkable. International donations are essential in making that commitment effective. It is possible that such donations have distorted health funding, making inefficient use of scarce resources for pharmaceutical purchases. These inefficiencies are however being corrected as the deepening economic crisis tests the ingenuity of the health system to protect the population from deteriorating standards of living.

Chapter 13: Health in a Survival Economy

"Good food, housing, money, and employment contribute to maintaining health...A garden, however small it may be, is better than a doctor."
(Alejandro Davila Bolanos, around 1960)

Health services may increase the length and improve the quality of people's lives, but their impact depends on the underlying economic and social environment. Before 1979 the chance to live a long, healthy life in Nicaragua was reserved for a privileged few. Among this group life expectancy was nearly as high as in the US or other industrialised countries. The poor majority, by contrast, were deprived not only of health care, but also of the other factors which play a role in health — food, land, income, safe water, sanitation, housing, education and other basic services.

The Sandinistas realised that the goal of 'health for all' could not be achieved simply by expanding the outreach of the health services. Fundamental changes in society were needed to narrow the health gap between the privileged few and the poor majority. These changes would entail, above all, a radical transformation of the country's economy.

But the economy was shattered as a result of the 18-month insurrection: factories, homes, hospitals, schools and public buildings had been destroyed or damaged by Somoza's National Guard. The total cost of the damage during the insurrection was estimated at $1.3 billion.[1] When the Sandinistas came to power they found only $3.5 million in the national treasury and faced a national debt of $1.6 billion.

The new Government decided to embark on a two-track policy of economic and social development. On the one hand, the economy would undergo a process of restructuring in order to distribute resources and opportunities more evenly. At the same time large-scale reconstruction would be encouraged to repair and rebuild the infrastructure needed for growth.[2]

The 'mixed' economy

One of the Government's first steps was to nationalise all property belonging to Somoza and his associates. This included one-fifth of all farm land, half the agro-processing industry, one-third of manufacturing capacity, and nearly all the fishing, forestry, mass transport and construction industries.[3] Foreign-owned assets in the mining and banana industries were also nationalised. In addition, the Government took control of banking and external trade, but limited expropriations of businesses and land outside the Somoza group. The Sandinistas stressed their commitment to a 'mixed' economy, in which the private sector would continue to play a leading role. Most business leaders and large landowners, however, deeply distrusted the Sandinistas and resented the Government's intervention in the economy.

Despite opposition from much of the business community, the early years of the Sandinista revolution were marked by unprecedented social progress and economic growth:

- Between 1979 and 1984 expenditure on education increased fourfold, the number of children attending primary school increased by 70%, and the number of school teachers doubled.[4]
- The population covered by social security rose from 200,000 to more than a million.[5]
- 300 new health posts and five hospitals were constructed.[6]
- 800 kilometres of new roads were built, including the first land route between the Pacific and the Atlantic Coasts.[7]
- Electricity was brought to 14,000 new users in rural areas.[8]
- 50,000 new telephone lines were installed, and direct telephone communication established with the Atlantic Coast for the first time.[9]
- Light industry grew rapidly, including food-processing (milk, vegetables, cooking oil, seafoods, sugar), clothing, pharmaceuticals, and leather goods.[10]
- New housing was built for 20,000 families.[11]
- New water supply systems reached 280,000 people in 450 communities; sanitary waste disposal reached 100,000 new users[12] (see Figure 13.1).

These developments were fuelled by large public expenditures made possible by loans from international banks, grants from UN-related organisations and East European Governments, and credit lines from West European and Latin American Governments. The introduction of a progressive tax system also obliged wealthy Nicaraguans to contribute to the country's social and economic development.

The quest for food security

The health of poor families depends, above all, on being able to grow enough food on their own land, or having the income to buy it. Before 1979, hunger was a daily fact of life for thousands of families. For the

Fig. 13.1

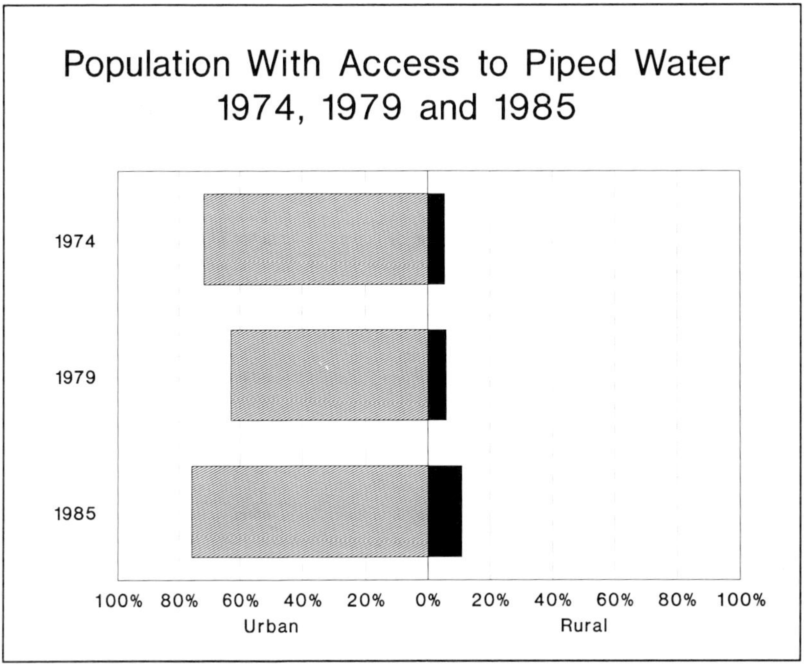

Only a modest increase in the proportion of the population with access to piped water has occurred.

poorest half of the population, average calorie availability was only about 80% of what was required for health.[13] In the poorest regions, only a third of the people had enough income to supply an adequate diet.[14] The richest 5%, by contrast, had enough food to meet 180% of their calorie needs.

One of the new Government's basic aims was to ensure that all social groups had enough food. Such a system of 'food security' would require radical changes in land ownership, agricultural production, food pricing and distribution. It would also have to pay special attention to the needs of the most vulnerable groups, especially low-income families.

When the Sandinistas came to power the country faced a major food deficit. The final months of the insurrection had severely disrupted the planting season in many parts of the country, resulting in sharp falls in the maize, beans and rice harvests. The Ministry of Agriculture moved fast to help small and medium-scale farmers. Before the revolution, 90% of credit for farmers had been used for export crops grown by large landowners. Now, for the first time, credit was made available to small and medium-scale farmers to grow food.[15] Between 1978 and 1981, the number of such farmers receiving credit rose from 23,158 to 80,455.[16]

Fig. 13.2

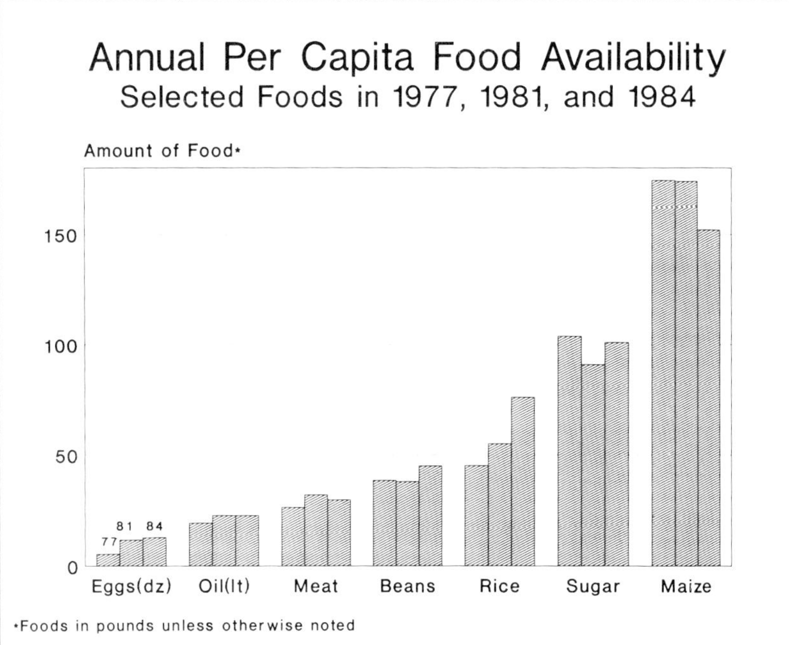

Despite rapid population growth, the availability of selected food items remained nearly constant throughout the early 1980s.

Another popular measure was a drastic reduction in rents on land used to grow food crops, and new institutions were created to provide farmers with technical assistance and a regular supply of seeds, fertilisers and other inputs. The National Basic Food Corporation, ENABAS, was established to guarantee minimum prices for food crops.

To meet the food deficit the Government was also obliged to import large quantities of maize and beans. Grain, milk, oil, and sugar were distributed as emergency rations. Food was also sold at subsidised prices through community stores, supermarkets, work place commissaries and canteens. Schools provided milk to students. Health clinics distributed food to pregnant and lactating women, and to families with malnourished children. The Ministry of Social Welfare started nurseries where the children of working parents were fed every day (see Chapter 9).

Emergency rations were phased out in 1980 and replaced by a system providing food supplements to families in need. By 1981 food availability was generally above pre-revolutionary levels (see Figure 13.2). Malnutrition was declining and it seemed that the nutritional rehabilitation units could soon be closed. A physician working in one of

Fig. 13.3

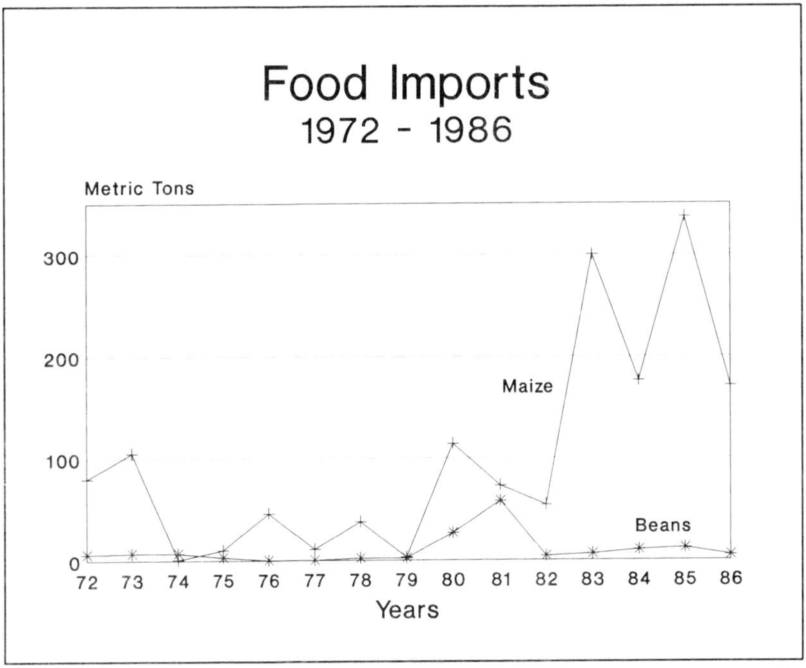

As production of food fell, imports were increasingly used to maintain availability.

these units commented, "These cases are left-overs of the past. Soon there will be no more."

The new agricultural policies had mixed results. In 1981 the bean crop was up, rice production was stagnant, and maize was down by 45%.[17] The great majority of Nicaraguans were eating much better than before the revolution, but at the cost of large food imports. This was a cost the Government could not afford indefinitely.

An already difficult situation was exacerbated when, in early 1981, the US abruptly suspended a wheat loan worth $9.6 million. This was the first of a series of economic sanctions aimed at crippling the economy and destabilising the Government.

In response, the Government launched the Nicaraguan Food Programme (PAN) in April 1981. PAN's central task was to ensure the supply of basic foods to the whole population by promoting the production of food crops by small and medium-scale farmers.[18] In the heady optimism of the days before the *Contra* war, government planners expected PAN to achieve national self-sufficiency in maize, rice and beans within three years. (Ironically, the Spanish word *pan* means 'bread', which could not be made without using imported wheat.)

The new programme concentrated mainly on helping peasant farmers through price incentives, credit, seeds, technical assistance, mechanised services, training, improved crop-storage facilities and transport. To overcome dependence on imported wheat, the Government promoted the use of maize. Festivals were organised involving recipe competitions, songs, and dance, all based on the theme *El maiz, nuestra raiz* ('Maize, our roots').

Self-sufficiency in basic foods, however, proved elusive. Torrential rains on the Pacific coast washed away the first maize crop of 1982. Those farmers who managed to replant were then ruined by a prolonged drought. Meanwhile, public demand for maize rose rapidly due to the growing population, heavily subsidised food prices, and the use of maize as a substitute for sorghum in animal feed. In 1983 the country faced a massive shortfall in maize which was covered by record imports (see Figure 13.3). Drastic measures were needed to boost production of the country's major food grain.

The Government responded by making large investments in maize production on state land.[19] Irrigated lands in the fertile Pacific region, normally used to grow cotton, were instead planted with maize for part of the year. As a result, the amount of maize grown on state farms almost doubled between 1982/83 and 1983/84. Yet it still accounted for only 14% of total maize production. And because it relied on imported equipment, state-produced maize was much more expensive than maize grown by peasants. The Farmers' and Ranchers' Organisation (UNAG) condemned the policy because it absorbed finance, equipment and expertise which otherwise could have been used to boost peasant food production.

Land to the tiller

The inauguration of PAN was followed in late 1981 by the Government's long-promised Agrarian Reform Law. This was potentially the single most important step toward boosting food production. Nicaragua has relatively abundant agricultural land, with an average of 23.7 hectares per rural family. (In nearby El Salvador, by contrast, the average is only 3.5 hectares per family.) Before the revolution, however, this land was divided very unevenly. In 1978 about 3,000 large farms accounted for nearly half the total agricultural land. Situated on the fertile plains of the Pacific region and using modern agricultural technology, these farms produced mainly export crops such as cotton, sugar and tobacco. Their owners (2% of the agricultural work force) also dominated bank credit facilities and technical assistance.

The other half of the country's farmland was dominated by small and medium-scale producers, who accounted for one-third of the rural work force. These farmers produced 70% of the country's main staple foods —

maize and beans — yet received little government credit or other assistance. Another 36% of rural families were poor farmers owning only 2% of the land, receiving no government assistance, and usually unable to grow enough food for their needs. The other one-third were either salaried or seasonal workers owning no land at all, and living in conditions of abject poverty.[20]

The new agrarian law was moderate in scope. Properties of over 300 hectares in the Pacific region and over 700 hectares elsewhere could be expropriated. Below this level, expropriation could be applied only to inefficient farmers, or those who maintained semi- feudal land tenure and labour relations. The law allowed for land to be distributed to peasant cooperatives, individual families and indigenous communities. In practice, the Ministry of Agriculture (MIDINRA) favoured cooperative ownership, rather than individual land titles.

Disincentives to production

While MIDINRA tried to boost food production, other government policies were having the unintended effect of actually discouraging farmers from producing food crops. One disincentive to farmers was the lack of consumer goods and farming tools at government-controlled shops in rural areas. Through their trade unions, farmers and farm workers complained bitterly that there were insufficient shops and that those in existence did not stock the machetes, rubber boots, kerosene, clothes, shoes and household goods which they wanted. Said one farmers' leader: "What's the point of working all year only to sell our products at low prices, and then not be able to find or buy what we need to clothe, feed and look after our families?"

Food subsidies were another disincentive to grain production. In order to provide enough basic foods to the urban poor and landless farm workers, the Government 'froze' food prices from 1981 onwards. This was achieved through massive consumer subsidies. Television commercials explained how ENABAS purchased maize at the relatively low rate of 1.8 *cordobas* a pound and sold it to the consumer for only one *cordoba* a pound — the difference, plus the cost of transport, packaging, drying and storage, being paid by the Government. A similar system applied to items such as beans, milk, flour, cooking oil, and even lettuces imported from Costa Rica.

It became cheaper for many farmers to buy food from the Government than to grow it themselves.[21] Many small-scale farmers stopped growing maize and beans and sought work in the cities instead. Large cotton and sugar estates stopped planting maize and beans for their workers. Instead, even state farms bought these items at subsidised prices.

The bubble bursts

Despite price and marketing problems, the production of basic foods gradually increased. The 1983/84 rice and bean crops reached record levels and maize production exceeded 500,000 metric tons for the first time since 1978/79.[22] Available calories were 40% higher than pre-revolutionary levels. Eating habits also changed. People ate less beef but more rice, maize, chicken and eggs than before the revolution (see Figure 13.2).

The overall economic outlook was still hopeful. In contrast to the other four Central American nations, the economy was still expanding: in 1983 the economy grew by 5%.[23] The cost of living was also lower in Nicaragua than anywhere else in the region, due largely to heavy government subsidies on food and items such as kerosene, soap and cooking oil. About 24,000 families had received land through the Agrarian Reform Law — either as members of cooperatives or individually — and were using it to grow food. Although government expenditure had increased enormously since 1979, inflation was still modest.

Most people seemed to approve of the policies of the Sandinista Government. In November 1984, the FSLN won 68% of the popular vote in the country's first general election since the end of the Somoza era.

But the bubble was about to burst. Nicaragua could no longer escape the consequences of the world economic recession, mounting external debts, and falling prices for its agricultural products. A massive trade

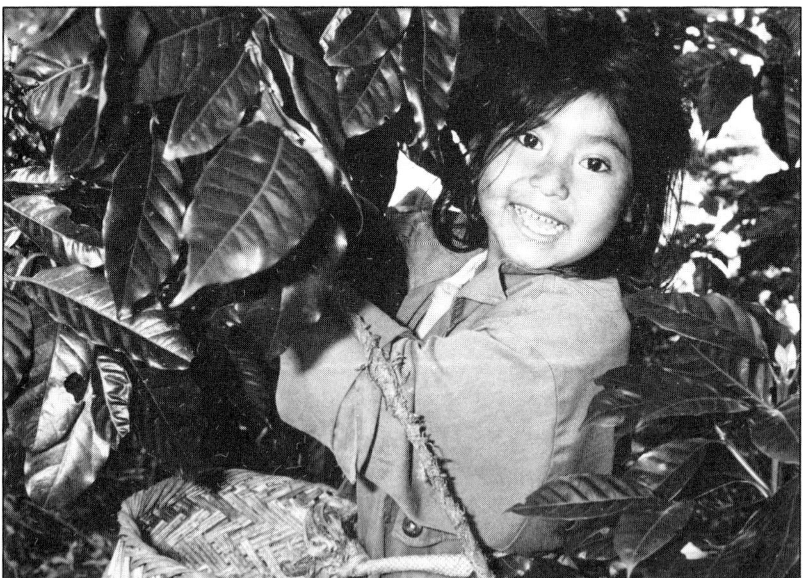

ANA CECILIA GONZALES

Harvesting coffee, Nicaragua's main export crop. Coffee production has been severely hit by the *Contra* war.

deficit placed the economy under intolerable strain. In 1984 Nicaragua imported goods worth $826 million, but the value of the country's exports was only $386 million.

Nicaragua also faced special problems because of the war. *Contra* targets included cooperatives, private farms and plantations, coffee processing plants, grain silos, power stations, ports, sawmills, trucks and buses, ambulances, health centres, schools, and children's nurseries and feeding centres. In 1984 about 120,000 people left their farms to seek safety in cities or special settlements, resulting in a sharp fall in the area planted with maize and beans.

The coffee harvest — which provided 60% of export revenue — was also severely hit because pickers could not move safely in many of the mountainous areas where the *Contras* operated. In the 1984/85 coffee harvest, more than 200 pickers were murdered by *Contra* forces and production valued at $69 million (one-fifth of total exports) was lost.

At the same time, intense lobbying by the US Government led to the denial of access to important regional and international sources of finance and development aid. The Governments of the UK and West Germany also sharply reduced or eliminated their aid. In May 1985 the US, which for decades had been Nicaragua's main trading partner, placed an embargo on most trade and commerce.

A 'survival' economy

By 1985 the Nicaraguan economy was in deep trouble. Production of food and cash crops fell, export income declined and inflation eroded the value of wages. People complained bitterly about shortages of food and consumer goods including chicken, powdered milk, eggs, cooking oil, toothpaste, toilet paper and light bulbs.

The Sandinistas responded by abandoning some of the policies they had pursued so whole-heartedly since coming to power. Proclaiming the need for a 'survival economy', they first set about reducing government expenditure, which was a prime contributing factor to the growing inflation.[24] Development projects, including roads, bridges, housing, sewerage and water supplies, were suspended. The budgets of nearly all government ministries were either frozen or cut. The only exceptions were health and defence, spending on both of which increased. Defence expenditure consumed about half the national budget.

The Government also took steps to boost the production of food and cash crops. Food subsidies, which had discouraged many farmers from planting maize and beans, were reduced.[25] This step was popular with farmers, but brought hardship to many urban poor and landless rural families who had to buy all or most of their food.

The Government ended the monopoly of ENABAS, allowing grain and bean producers to sell their crops to other buyers. Private cooperatives began to replace state enterprises in the sale of agricultural tools, basic foods and consumer goods in rural areas. In the department of Esteli, for example, the local branch of the farmers' organisation UNAG established a network of shops selling items such as boots, shirts, seeds, kerosene, tools and clothing. The larger shops also served as storage and marketing centres, helping small farmers and cooperatives to market their crops more efficiently. A local UNAG president said: "The best incentive policy is one where the producers can get medicine for their animals, where the workers can get boots, trousers and shorts, where there are medicines for our children, and where goods produced in the cities reach the countryside at prices the *campesinos* can afford."

The Government also decided to accelerate the pace of agrarian reform and to reduce the emphasis on collective agriculture. Between 1984 and 1986 about 74,000 rural families received land — 60% individually and the remainder via cooperatives. In early 1986 the Agrarian Reform Law was amended to permit the expropriation of underutilised private farms without regard to size.

By the end of 1986, Nicaragua's agrarian structure had changed profoundly. Two million hectares of farmland (40% of the total) had been distributed to 98,000 families, either individually or through cooperatives.[26] Large-scale farmers owned only one-fifth of all farmland, compared with half in 1978 (see Figure 13.4). About 40% of the rural

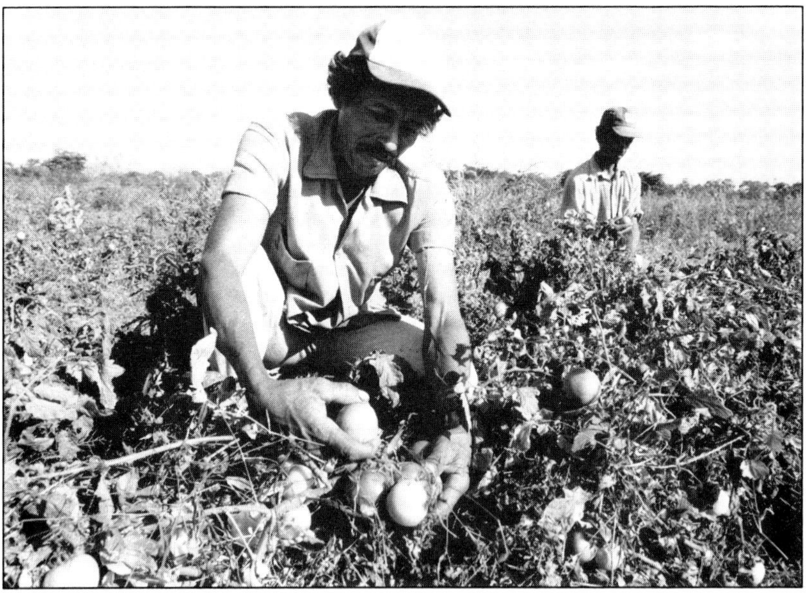

MIKE GOLDWATER

Farmers harvest tomatoes at the Fanor Urroz Cooperative, on the Rio Grande, near Managua. The cooperative received its land from the Government after further expropriation of large land holdings in 1985.

Fig. 13.4

Land Tenure
Size/Type of Agricultural Holdings

Type of Ownership	1978	1986
State Farms	0	13%
Full Cooperatives	0	13%
<35 Hectares, not in Coop	17%	12%
<35 Hectares, in Coop	1%	10%
35 - 141 Hectares, Private	30%	30%
>141 Hectares, Private	52%	22%

Source: Barraclough SL, Scott MF, *The rich have already eaten*, London: Transnational Institute, 1987.

population had received land through the agrarian reform. Landless labourers were still 25% of the rural work force, but many more had year-round employment and the benefits of membership in the agricultural workers' union.

Economic and military attacks focused the attention of Sandinista leaders on economic and political survival. Ironically, the result was increased privatisation of agricultural production and services via individual holdings and cooperatives, rather than greater control by central government. The effects on production were soon evident: in 1986/87 the maize harvest was well above the pre-revolutionary levels, rice production doubled, and bean production reached a new record (see Figure 13.5).

Protecting the poor

Agrarian reform was an essential step in reaching food security, but it was not enough. Special measures were needed to ensure that the most vulnerable — especially the urban poor and landless farm workers — also had enough food. This was the purpose of the 'guarantee card' system introduced in 1982. Intended originally to distribute sugar more evenly,

Fig. 13.5

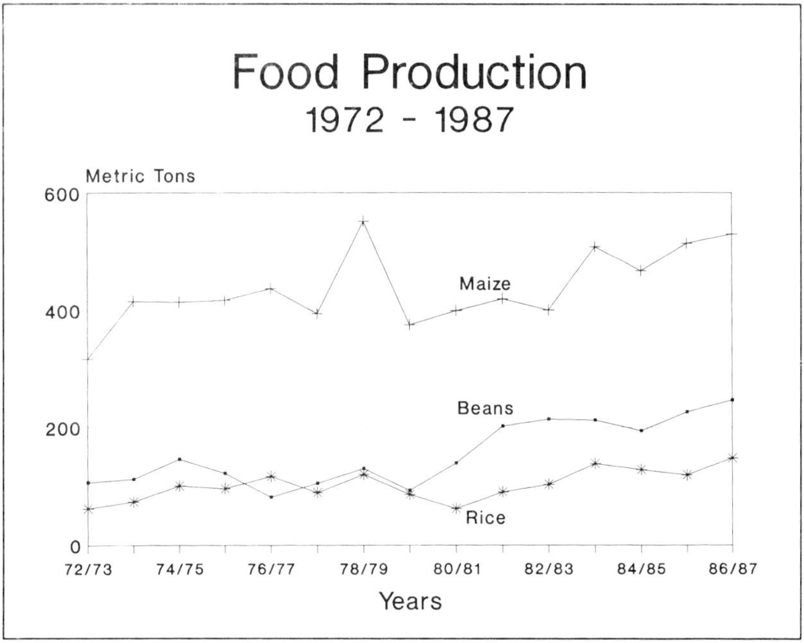

the system was later extended to cover rice, beans, cooking oil and soap, which were sold at subsidised rates through community shops.[27] The system made these items widely available. Even more important, it helped hundreds of thousands of poor families to meet their basic living expenses.

But with the escalation of the *Contra* war and the deterioration of the economy, the guarantee card system was gradually whittled away. By early 1988 the Government could guarantee only one kilo of sugar, a half-kilo of rice, and one bar of soap per household every month.

1988 — 'the worst year'

As the Nicaraguan revolution approached its tenth anniversary, the country faced a crippling economic crisis compounded by eight years of war. At the start of 1988 the Government declared a state of food emergency after a severe drought wiped out 75% of the bean crop, 45% of sorghum production, and 25% of the maize harvest. Said Henry Ruiz, Minister of Economic Cooperation:[28]

"Food security is not a question of balancing proteins and calories. It's a question of having enough rice and beans to last out the war."

The economy was now in desperate shape. Export revenues plummeted to about $200 million annually, a decline of 30% from pre-

Fig. 13.6

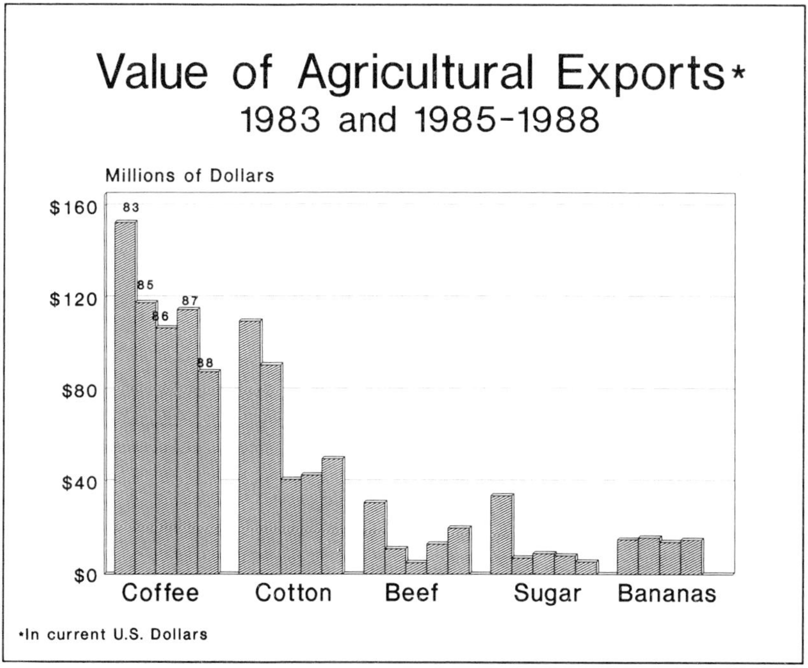

The value of most agricultural exports declined seriously in the late 1980s.

revolution levels (see Figure 13.6). The national debt reached $7 billion, the highest per capita debt in Latin America. Foreign aid and credits reached a high of $1.2 billion in 1985; they fell to $385 million in 1987. Galloping inflation reduced economic planning to guesswork. Real wages in 1988 had lost 94% of their value compared with 1980[29] (see Figure 13.7).

The impact of the war on agriculture and the economy as a whole has been devastating. More than 278,000 hectares of agricultural land have been abandoned by peasants seeking safety from *Contra* attacks, reducing the production of food and export crops. Between 1984 and 1987 the country lost the equivalent of 40% of export earnings through destroyed infrastructure and lost agricultural and industrial output. Direct destruction was valued at $222 million, while total losses (including lost production and the value of secondary industries) were estimated at $2.6 billion.

The war also had more insidious effects on the economy and health. With defence spending absorbing half the budget, all other sectors suffered. Routine maintenance of schools, water systems, health facilities, factories, government vehicles and equipment was neglected

Fig. 13.7

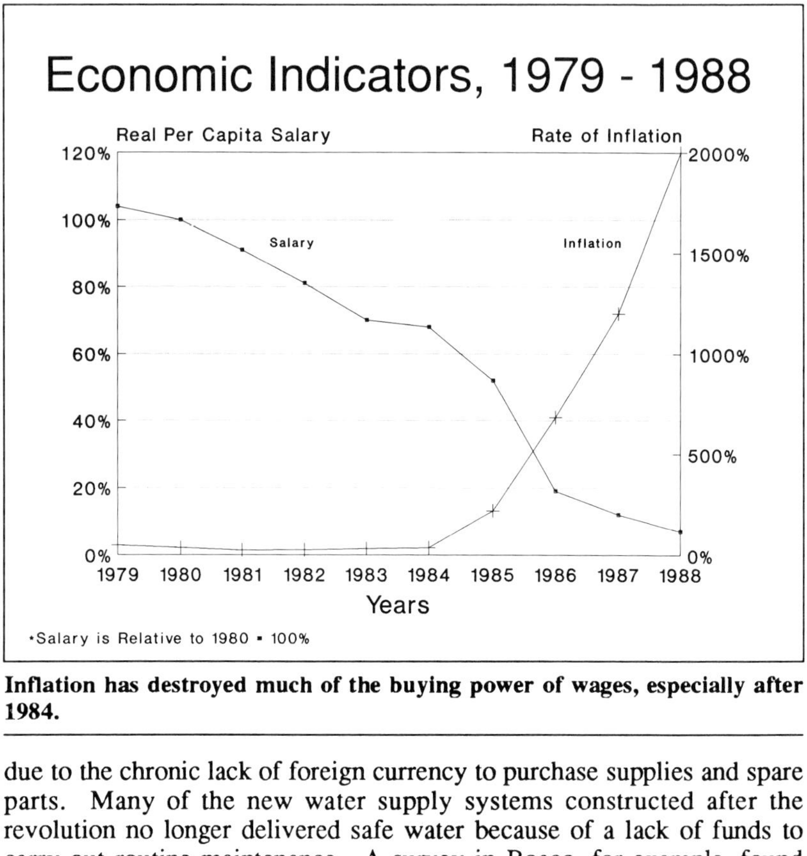

Inflation has destroyed much of the buying power of wages, especially after 1984.

due to the chronic lack of foreign currency to purchase supplies and spare parts. Many of the new water supply systems constructed after the revolution no longer delivered safe water because of a lack of funds to carry out routine maintenance. A survey in Boaco, for example, found that only a quarter of the rural water systems built after 1979 were still providing water of acceptable quality.[30] In Managua's slum neighbourhoods the combination of unsafe water, inadequate sanitation and heaps of fly-infested refuse produced favourable conditions for the spread of infection, especially diarrhoea. The collection of urban refuse was irregular or non-existent because of a lack of vehicles, tyres and spare parts.

In February 1988 the Government announced a 3,000% devaluation of the *cordoba* as part of a series of measures designed to check the downward slide of the economy. This was followed four months later by a package of economic measures which shocked many of the Government's own supporters by its severity. Aimed at reducing the trade deficit and boosting exports, the measures amounted to a conventional International Monetary Fund package without the financing

Fig. 13.8

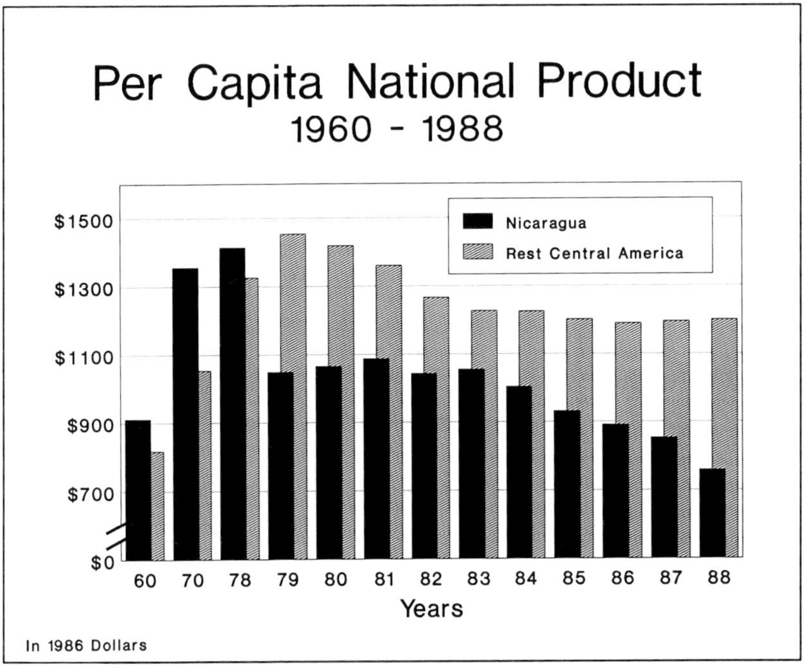

Nicaragua's per capita national product rose rapidly during the 1960s and 1970s. It declined sharply in the revolutionary insurrection of 1978 and 1979 and recovered moderately in the early 1980s, only to decline again during the *Contra* war of the late 1980s. This contrasts with the recession experienced by the rest of Central America during the early 1980s which was followed by a modest recovery during the late 1980s.

that accompanies IMF reforms. Price controls were lifted on almost all goods and services, and most subsidies were abolished. Rice and bean prices tripled, meat and fish prices doubled, petrol rose twelve-fold, cooking gas rose ten-fold and electricity rose seven-fold.

These measures slashed the purchasing power of wage earners. Government employees received some protection through the monthly distribution of five kilos of rice, five kilos of beans and three kilos of sugar. Low-income urban and rural workers also received salary increases enabling them to purchase 60% of a 'basket' of basic foods with their monthly salary.

Those least affected by these measures were food producers, who continued to receive government credit and could sell their rice, maize and beans on the free market. In the first half of 1988 a cease-fire and early rains also enabled farmers to plant 16,000 more hectares of maize and beans. The first rice, maize and bean crops of 1988 were well up on the previous year.

These harvests were followed, in October 1988, by the devastating hurricane 'Joan', which destroyed food and export crops, roads, electricity supplies, food processing plants, schools, health facilities and 30,000 homes.[31] Total damage was estimated at $840 million — four times the country's annual export earnings.

According to government economist Mario Arana, 1988 was "the worst of the revolution. In one year we lost all the achievements of the eight previous years." In December, inflation reached the incredible rate of 30,000%. Although all the Central American countries suffered recession throughout the 1980s, Nicaragua was by far the hardest hit (see Figure 13.8). Production fell by about 8% in 1988 and is expected to fall by a similar amount in 1989. The Nicaraguan Government estimates that per capita GDP has fallen to about $300 — lower even than that of Haiti, long the poorest country in the western hemisphere.

The future of the revolution now hinges on the ability of the Government to stimulate production and control inflation. A 30% cut in the Government's budget and a 117% devaluation in January 1989 reflected a bold attempt to control hyperinflation and stimulate the economy. Guaranteed food prices for consumers and most subsidies for producers were eliminated. The effects of these measures are hard to predict. A total of 20 devaluations were carried out between January and August 1989 in an effoert to reduce inflation. No one, however, expects these reforms to start to bear fruit until the early 1990s.

Chapter 14: The Nicaraguan Health Model

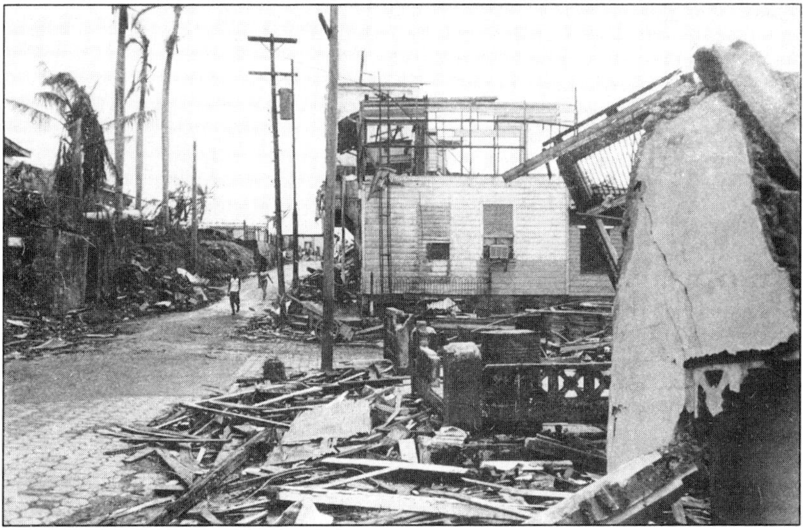

FRANK JUDD

Devastation in Bluefields, on the Atlantic Coast, caused by Hurricane Joan.

The most powerful hurricane to reach Central America in a century hit the Atlantic Coast town of Bluefields on 22 October 1988 and cut a swathe of destruction across the country. The damage was even greater than that caused by the 1972 earthquake, but the reaction to the disaster could not have been more different.[1]

In the hours before the hurricane half a million people were evacuated to safety. As a result of this quick action, the number of deaths was limited to 148. In the weeks which followed, the Bluefields sawmill worked all day, every day, even though half of its roof had collapsed. Teams of volunteers cleared the streets, piling up rubble every 20 feet. Despite a conspicuous lack of aid from all but a few countries, relief work was prompt and efficient. Thousands of people were provided with shelter in schools and other public buildings across the country. Three weeks later, only 800 people had not yet returned to rebuild their homes. Extensive health precautions were credited with preventing epidemics of diarrhoea and malaria..

Hurricane 'Joan' was only the most recent of many disasters to hit Nicaragua during the past two decades (see Figure 14.1). Yet despite two wars, a shattered economy, and a series of natural disasters, the Sandinistas have established and maintained a health system which meets the basic needs of most people. That system, for all its shortcomings, is

Fig. 14.1

Destruction in Five Disasters

Millions of Dollars*

Disaster	Damage to Health Facilities	Total Direct Damage
Earthquake, 1972	25	5400
Insurrection, 1978-1979	8	1300
Floods, 1982	18	420
Contra War, 1981-1984	6	222
Hurricane Joan, 1988	44	840

*in 1988 Dollars

Sources: Espinosa H, Murguia W, Perez E, 'La situacion de la salud en la economia Nicaraguense post-terremoto', Managua 1975, Masters' thesis, UNAN. ECLA, *Nicaragua: economic repercussions of recent political events*, Santiago de Chile: United Nations, 1979. ECLA, *Nicaragua: Las inundaciones de Mayo de 1982 u sus repercusiones sobre el desarrollo economico y social del pais*, Mexico: United Nations, 1982. INEC, *Efectos socio-economicos de la guerra de agresion*, Managua: INEC, 1988. ECLAC, *Report on damage caused to Nicaragua by hurricane Joan*, New York: United Nations, 1988.

eloquent testimony to the revolution's commitment to health for all.

Nicaragua began the 1980s as a middle-income developing country with an infant mortality rate characteristic of poorer developing countries. In the ten years since the revolution the infant mortality rate has fallen sharply[2] but income levels have also plummeted. Much of the improvement in infant mortality and other health benefits are in large part the result of government-initiated programmes. Further health improvements will depend on a better economy and improved living standards, and will require expanded involvement of the health system in preventive community health activities.[3]

The national agenda

The Government has adopted a variety of flexible approaches in an attempt to build a 'pluralist' form of socialism in the 1980s. These approaches include a mixed economy and decentralised administration —

characteristics more common among social democratic governments in industrialised countries. Developing countries such as Nicaragua, however, suffer from a chronic shortage of capital for investment in social and economic development.[4] The US decision to try to destroy the Sandinista Government has made this capital shortage far worse.

To manage and mobilise resources, socialist governments in developing countries, including China and Cuba, nationalised their economies. By the 1980s this model had lost much of its appeal, having led to the development of a privileged bureaucratic elite and condemned both countries to isolation from potential markets, sources of capital, and modern technology.

During the 1980s, revolutionary governments have looked for models which might generate less social dislocation and more rapid economic growth. Nicaragua and Zimbabwe are prime exponents of a more moderate road toward socialism.[5] The strategy has paid off for both countries, albeit in limited ways. Providing loans and credits to the private sector in Nicaragua stimulated the economy in the early 1980s and may have reduced or delayed hostile acts, including a possible direct US military intervention. But this moderate, mixed public-private road toward socialism led to a more capital-intensive, doctor-based health system than might otherwise have occurred.

The health agenda

Health has been a high priority in the Sandinista political agenda at least since the elaboration of the 'Historic Programme of the FSLN' in 1969.[6] That agenda proposed to 'empower' people to identify their health needs, organise them to realise their health goals, and involve them in the institutions and programmes which developed. The original agenda was not influenced by the strategy of primary health care, which was elaborated a decade later at Alma Ata. It has sometimes evolved in unexpected ways. Sandinista Government plans have often been modified under pressure from doctors, community groups, or other ministries. Increasingly, financial limitations and growing demands for care have led to an approach which is guided by a primary health care orientation in the choice of technologies, services and target populations.

In the early years of the revolution, health programmes which increased access to hospital care and medicines responded well to people's felt needs.[7] The health system was living testimony that the revolutionaries had made good their promises. It also created expectations that the system was unable to meet. The 'have-nots' rapidly became enthusiastic consumers of modern health services. Yet while people could be mobilised for massive, government-led campaigns, they were often not sufficiently 'empowered' to develop and direct day-to-day services. To many pro-FSLN activists, involvement in health campaigns became an expression of faith in the revolution and loyalty to the government. Attempts at further health reform seemed to question that faith.

Like socialist revolutionaries in other countries,[8] the Sandinistas went through two stages in developing health services. The first was a rapid expansion in coverage of conventional care, responding to pre-revolutionary goals and plans. The second was a reformulation of health plans in response to the economic, political and social environment. Some countries, such as the USSR during the New Economic Plan in the 1920s, did this under conditions of extreme scarcity. Others, such as Cuba with its community medicine programme starting in 1976, did it in relative affluence. Nicaragua reformulated its health system between 1983 and 1986 in response to scarcity and war, without nationalisation or affluence.

Investing in health

Ten years before the Sandinistas came to power, Costa Rica began to invest heavily in health services. Twenty years earlier, Cuba had begun a new health system with the advent of its socialist revolution.[9] In each country, expanded services and improved health were apparent within a decade (see Figure 14.2). Costa Rica was also able to build on 60 years of investments in education and development infrastructure. Cuban resources were mobilised through nationalisation and Soviet assistance. The changes in Nicaragua have been no less dramatic, despite worse underlying health conditions and far more limited resources.

Sandinista supporters often point to the rapid expansion of the health system in the early 1980s as one of the revolution's outstanding achievements. The reorganisation in the late 1980s, however, may well be a more useful example for other developing countries.

Large investments in modern health services cannot be sustained in a developing country with a deteriorating economy. This became apparent in Nicaragua in 1983, when economic realities forced the Government to re-evaluate the health system it had built. To continue the doctor-run, hospital-based programmes of the early 1980s would effectively have excluded many people from the system. The numbers of medical visits and supervised births were already declining by 1984. A new approach was needed which would provide services more efficiently and generate additional resources for the health system.

Examples of the new approach emerged clearly by 1988. They included the 'Campaign to Defend the Lives of Children', the '*barrio* doctor' programme, and new roles for health volunteers and traditional birth attendants. These were remarkably moderate responses to a political situation which might have provoked more radical actions, such as the nationalisation of all health resources. While the Sandinistas armed the people to defend socialism, they also strengthened the conditions for private medical practice.

Despite the revolution in primary health care which started in Alma

Fig. 14.2

Cuba, Costa Rica and Nicaragua on the Eve of Change and 7 Years Later

	Cuba		Costa Rica		Nicaragua	
	1959	1966	1969	1976	1979	1986
Doctors per 10,000 Population	9.0	8.5	5.6	6.6	5.0	5.4
Infant Mortality Rate	62	40	69	28	90	76
Life Expectancy at Birth	63	68	65	70	55	60
Diarrhoea Deaths per 100,000 Population	70	20	130	19	*200	*100
Beds per 10,000 Population	42	47	40	35	18	15
Percent of Births Attended	63	78	70	82	37	40
Medical Visits Per Capita	2.0	2.8	2.0	2.9	0.8	2.3

*Estimated

Sources: Danielson R, *Cuban medicine*, New Brunswick: Transaction Books, 1979. Mohs E, 'Infectious diseases and health in Costa Rica: the development of a new paradigm,' *Paediatric Infectious Disease* 1982; 3: 212-5. Saenz L, *Salud sin riqueza: el caso de Costa Rica*, San Jose: Ministerio de Salud, 1985.

Ata in 1978, the gap between health 'haves' and 'have-nots' has generally widened, according to World Health Organisation Director Hiroshi Nakajima.[10] But in Nicaragua this gap has narrowed. To achieve this, many components of the health system have been limited, cut back, or reorganised. What is left in towns, neighbourhoods, and villages throughout the country is a health service which is more modest and more sustainable.

Investments in medicines, doctors, and hospitals are less effective in improving the quality of life than spending on food, latrines, and basic education. Expansion of health services, however, visibly responds to the desires of the people and the interests of the government. Myrna Cunningham, physician and governor of Northern Zelaya, observed:[11]

"Many things the revolution would like to do are slow. You can't build a road or make good nutrition overnight. But health is something you can do in every village, and right away. It is a way for the revolution to get to everybody, anywhere in Nicaragua."

Investments in health care also make sense as part of the government's long-range strategy. Some improvement in health would no doubt arise from sustained, balanced economic growth. The Sandinistas have not yet been able to mobilise adequate resources or control the conditions of the economy. They have, however, mobilised more modest resources and coordinated non-public resources to provide health care. Such care provides a safety net to protect the population from some of the threats to health which result from the decline in living conditions. It also provides a much needed point of unity to reduce political polarisation.

The Nicaraguan model

The Nicaraguan health system today is an eclectic mix of elements. Special features of this model include mixed public/private services, the participation of community organisations in dealing with a wide variety of problems, large-scale health education efforts, an extensive rural primary health network staffed by social service physicians, and underfunded and overused hospitals. These diverse components make up 'territorial health systems' around the country. These components must be carefully coordinated by MINSA to build the health system in the decade ahead.

International participation in the system is widespread. It includes European volunteers who staff church and government clinics, solidarity committees which collect equipment and medicines to supply health facilities, and bilateral and multilateral programmes to build and run hospitals, train and equip traditional birth attendants, and supply nutritional supplements.

Small-scale donations from religious and political groups in the US, for example, provide a quarter of the operating budget of the national children's hospital. From 1981 to 1985, Cuban physicians provided 24% of all public medical consultations in the country.[12] The Swiss, East German, Soviet, Dutch, and Norwegian Governments have each built or are currently running hospitals. "But even more than the money," says Health Minister Dora Maria Tellez, "we depend on international solidarity for human values and the experience that people bring. This is their revolution, too." At least five foreign health workers are among the more than thirty *internacionalistas* killed in the *Contra* war so far.

The efficiency of investments in health has improved. Primary care began with plans for comprehensive services, formalised in the 18

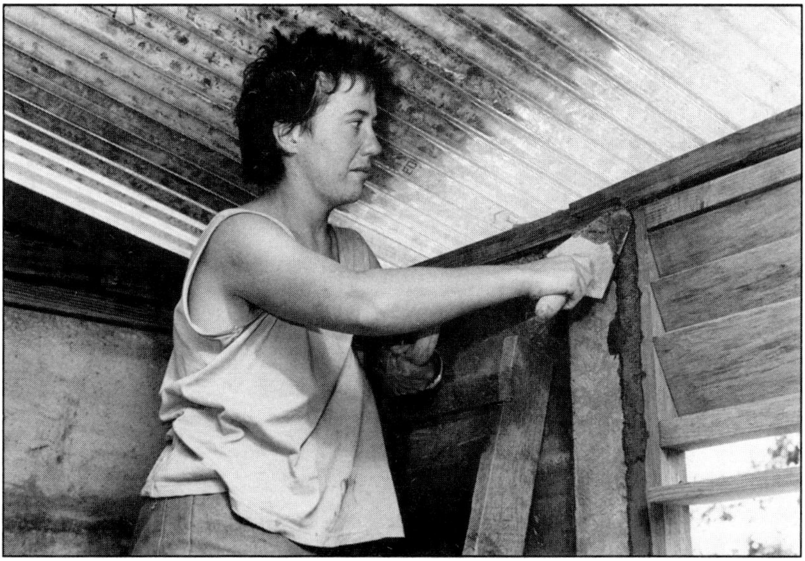

ANA CECILIA GONZALES

Thousands of volunteers from all over the world come to Nicaragua, including manual workers, qualified health workers and other professionals. This volunteer is helping to build a school and a health centre at the Cooperative Ignacio Ramon Olivas, near Matagalpa.

programmes of PIASS. Step by step, these lofty goals have been revised. Programmes for universal coverage have been restricted to focus on groups at special risk, especially pregnant women, and children under five years of age. Priorities have been trimmed to focus primarily on the major causes of preventable death, including diarrhoea, respiratory disease, violence and accidents. Health education has been given precedence over more costly strategies of improved sanitation, water supply, and nutrition.

The Nicaraguan primary care system hardly represents the 'selective' strategy which some experts advocate for primary care in poor countries.[13] The 'selective' model usually involves a package of services provided in a uniform manner by national-level administrators. The services are not easily revised or adapted to local situations. By contrast, the Nicaraguan approach has evolved mainly from local needs and interests. It is administered regionally or sub-regionally via 'territorial health systems', and depends on decisions and resources which are generated in part from local offices of government ministries and community organisations. The Nicaraguan approach to limitations in primary care is now receiving its most severe test in the 'Campaign to Defend the Lives of Children'. One example of MINSA's role in coordinating multisectoral resources is the encouragement of women's groups to petition their cooperatives to reserve the milk of a cow for pregnant and lactating women.

During the past decade, 31 poor countries with a combined population of one billion people have suffered sustained declines in health.[14] In Latin America alone, it is estimated that 130 million people lack access to basic modern health services. Primary health care in such areas demands "new forms of dialogue between communities, health professionals, and social and political groups..."[15] This book highlights a decade of such dialogue.

Nicaragua today has a *de facto* two-tier health system. In rural areas, services are provided mainly at public facilities staffed by professionals doing social service, local auxiliary staff, or volunteers with a medical bag. The options in urban areas include public and private doctors, health centres, pharmacies and hospitals.

In both the urban and rural areas, coordination between primary and secondary care has proved difficult. For problems including diarrhoea, giving birth and cervical cancer, a good mix of simple curative and specialised back-up services has evolved. Other problems, including nutrition, abortion, and respiratory diseases, are still dealt with in a more haphazard and less effective manner.

The unique power of doctors to make or break this system has become apparent. Nicaragua is still producing doctors with a curative, clinical orientation.[16] The health of groups still seems less important than the treatment of an individual case. MINSA has attempted to placate organised medicine by instituting only limited reforms in medical schools and hospitals. An unintended result of this approach has been to limit the potential of preventive medicine and community health efforts. Until medical education undergoes further reform, the prevention of diarrhoea and malnutrition are likely to receive less attention than their treatment.

In 1979 the FSLN declared that health care was a right of the people and a responsibility of the government. The war and economic decline have forced a change in this philosophy. According to Health Minister Tellez, "It is still the responsibility of the Government to provide health care, but only to the degree that the people demonstrate a willingness to take part. Health is a shared responsibility of the government and people. Our responsibility is to respond to peoples' concerns and focus their resources."

Recovery and development

Will Nicaragua be able to rebuild its shattered economy and heal the wounds in its divided society in the wake of the *Contra* war? The answer depends, in part, on the capacity of the Sandinistas to defuse social and political tensions and achieve a large measure of national reconciliation. It also depends on the attitudes of local opposition leaders and former *Contra* rebels returning to their homeland to take part in civilian life once more.

But to a large extent the answer also depends on Washington. The

United States still exerts overwhelming political and economic influence in Central America. If the US Government continues to isolate Nicaragua, the prospects for national reconciliation and development may well be bleak. Professionals and technicians will continue to leave the country and only limited amounts of international aid will be available.

As this book goes to press, the prospects for peace in Nicaragua appear brighter than at any time in the past eight years. The five Central American Presidents have reached an agreement for the *Contras* to be disbanded. In return, the Nicaraguan Government has made important concessions to the internal opposition. But even if the fighting stops, Nicaragua will still be confronted with an economic and social crisis of daunting proportions. Whatever Government takes power after the elections in February 1990 will face an enormous reconstruction bill, estimated at $3 billion, in the context of an ailing economy and a deteriorating infrastructure.

Nicaragua has become a very poor country and badly needs international development assistance. Many Western Governments, however, still take much the same line as the United States and give little or no economic aid to Nicaragua. The UK Government, for example, gives no direct bilateral assistance, and the aid given by the European Community consists largely of food aid. If the EC were to give more financial and technical aid and also use its influence to persuade the US to lift its embargo on trade and credit, Nicaraguans would have more hope of rebuilding their shattered economy and reducing the tensions in their highly polarised society.

This book has described the processes of change and development in Nicaragua's health system during the 1980s, showing how the revolution's early ideals of comprehensive, free health provision have evolved to more modest aims of effective, targeted primary health care. The commitment to basic, universally available health care, as a shared responsibility of the government and the people, remains unchanged. The future of Nicaragua's unique experiment in primary health care now depends largely on the response of the international community to the opportunities emerging from the imminent end of the *Contra* war.

NOTES AND REFERENCES

Abbreviations Used in the Text

ADN	Nicaraguan Demographic Association
AMNLAE	Louisa Amanda Espinosa Women's Association
APHA	American Public Health Association
ATC	Rural Workers' Association
BCN	Banco Central de Nicaragua
CAHI	Central American Historical Institute
CAM	Centre for Medical Supplies (MINSA)
CARE	Citizens Active in Relief Everywhere
CDS	Sandinista Defence Committees
CELADE	Latin American Demographic Centre
CEPAD	Evangelical Committee for Aid and Development
CEPAL	Latin American Centre for Population Studies
CIES	Centre for Health Information and Studies
CIERA	Centre for Information and Studies of the Agrarian Reform
CPS	Popular Health Councils
DECOPS	Office for Popular Health Education and Communication (MINSA)
DINEI	National Division for Statistics and Information (MINSA)
ECLAC	Economic Commission for Latin America and the Caribbean
FSLN	Sandinista Front for the Liberation of Nicaragua
FETSALUD	Federation of Health Workers
JGN	National Government of Reconstruction
IADB	Inter-American Development Bank
INEC	National Institute for Studies and Censuses
INSSBI	National Institute for Social Security and Social Welfare
MIFIN	Ministry of Finance
MIDINRA	Ministry of Agrarian Reform
MINSA	Ministry of Health
MIPLAN	Ministry of Planning
OAS	Organisation of American States
OPS	Pan American Health Organisation
OMS	World Health Organisation
OXFAM	Oxford Committee for Famine Relief
PAHO	Pan American Health Organisation
PAN	National Food Programme
UNAG	National Farmers' Union
UNAN	National Autonomous University
UNESCO	United Nations Education and Cultural Organisation
UNICEF	United Nations Children's Fund
USAID	United States Agency for International Development
USHEW	United States Department of Health, Education, and Welfare
WHO	World Health Organisation

Organisations Which Coordinate Medical Assistance to Nicaragua

Scottish Medical Aid Campaign
c/o Volunteer Centre, 25/27 Elmbank Street, Glasgow, UK

Nicaragua Health Fund
c/o Sarah Jackson, 83 Margaret Street, London, England W1N 7HB

National Central America Health Rights Network
853 Broadway, Room 416, New York, NY 10003 212-420-9635

Association Medicale pour l'amerique latine et les caribes
c/o Raymond Herrera, CP 458, Station H, Montreal, Quebec, Canada H3G 2L1

Gesundheitsbrigade Schweiz-Nicaragua
c/o Zentralamerikasekretariat, Baslerstrasse 106, CH-8048 Zurich, Switzerland

Comitato solidarieta medica con il Nicaragua,
Casella postale 2536, CH-6500 Bellinzona, Switzerland

COBRISA (Brigada de Salud Aleman)
c/o Gesundheitsladen Berlin, D-1 Berlin 61, Germany

Nicaragua Health Aid,
G.P.O. 5421CC, Melbourne, Vic. 3001, Australia

REFERENCES

Preface

1 Nicaragua Health Study Collaborative at Harvard, CIES, UNAN, 'Health effects of the war in two rural communities in Nicaragua', *American Journal of Public Health* 1989; 79(4): 424-9.

Chapter 1

1 Espinosa H, Murguia W, Perez E, 'La situacion de la salud en la economia Nicaraguense post-terremoto', Managua 1975, Masters' thesis, UNAN. *see also*: Vijil C, 'The earthquake in Managua', *The Lancet* 1973; 1: 146.
2 ECLA, *Nicaragua: economic repercussions of recent political events*, Santiago de Chile: United Nations, 1979.
3 Rosset P, Vandermeer J, eds, *Nicaragua: unfinished revolution*, New York: Grove Press, 1986. *see also*: Vilas CM, *Perfiles de la revolucion Sandinista*, Buenos Aires: Editorial Legasa, 1984.
4 Equipo interdisciplinario latinoamericano, *Teoria y practica revolucionaria en Nicaragua*, Managua: Ediciones Contemporaneas, 1983.
5 Conroy M, *Nicaragua, profiles of the revolutionary public sector*, Boulder: Westview Press, 1987.
6 UNICEF/WHO Joint Committee on Health, *National decision-making for primary health care*, Geneva: WHO, 1981.

7 Chavez R, 'Urban planning in Nicaragua, the first five years', *Latin American Perspectives* 1987; 14(2): 226-36.
8 Wilson PA, 'Regionalization and decentralization in Nicaragua', *Latin American Perspectives* 1987; 14(2):237-54.
9 IADB, *Economic and social progress in Latin America*, Washington, DC: IADB, 1977.
10 Garfield RM, Rodriguez PF, 'Health and health services in Central America', *Journal of the American Medical Association* 1985; 254: 936-43.
11 Chavez R, *op. cit.*

Chapter 2

1 The Rector at the time was Carlos Tummerman, who later became Minister of Education and subsequently Ambassador to the United States.
2 MINSA/FETSALUD, 'Los trabajadores de la salud, su lucha historica y su participacion en las jornadas populares de salud', *Primer Congreso Nacional JPS*, Managua: MINSA, 1984.
3 Bolanos AD, *El interrogatorio*, Masaya: Libreria Loaisiga, 1979.
4 *ibid.*
5 Fox RW, Huguet JW, *Population and urban trends in Central America and Panama*, Washington DC: Inter-American Development Bank, 1977.
6 Escudero JC, 'Starting from year one: the politics of health in Nicaragua', *International Journal of Health Services* 1980; 10(4): 647-56.
7 Nunez O, 'Las politicas de salud del estado en Nicaragua: sobre-explotacion, deterioro fisico-mental de la fuerza de trabajo y reserva infantil de mano de obra', *Congreso Centroamericano de Sociologia 1978*, Tegucigalpa, Honduras, 1978.
8 JGN, *La salud en Nicaragua antes y despues del de la revolucion*, Managua: MINSA, 1980.
9 Halperin D, Garfield R, 'Developments in health care in Nicaragua', *New England Journal of Medicine* 1982; 307: 388-92.
10 Tefel RA, Mendoza H, Flores J, 'Social welfare', In: Walker T, ed, *Nicaragua: The first five years*, New York: Praeger, 1985.
11 USAID, *Health sector assessement for Nicaragua*, Managua: USAID Mission, 1976.
12 USDHEW, *Syncrisis: the dynamics of health*, Publication No. (OS) 74-50007, Washington, DC: USGPO, 1978.
13 Saenz L, *Integracion y coordinacion de los servicios de salud de Centroamerica*, San Salvador: ODECA, 1971.
see also: Paredes JA, *Los recursos de la salud publica en Centro America*, San Salvador: ODECA, 1968.
14 USAID, *op. cit.*
15 *ibid.*
16 MINSA/FETSALUD, 'Los trabajadores de la salud, su lucha historica y su participacion en las jornadas populares de salud', *Primer Congreso Nacional JPS*, Managua: MINSA, 1984.
17 Kuhl CA, *Report on the health situation in Nicaragua to the 33rd World Health Assembly*, Managua: MINSA, 1980.
18 Cabezas O, *Fire from the mountain*, New York: Crown Publishers, 1985.
19 Bollag U, 'Utilization of local first aiders in the provision of health care for

prisoners by the International Committee of the Red Cross in Nicaragua', *Journal of Community Health* 1985; 10(1): 17-21.
20 Zembrana DR, Huertas P, 'Aportes para la comprension del comportamiento del sistema de salud en el marco de las guerras populares de liberacion', *Revista Centroamericana de Ciencias de la Salud* 1980; 17: 135-42.
21 MINSA, 'Que es el sistem nacional unico de salud?' *Circular No.1*, Managua: MINSA, 1980.
22 'Brigada medica Cubana a Puerta Cabezas', *MINSA Boletin Informativa 6*, 10/24/79.
23 'Sera gigantesca labor de salud', *Barricada* 8/5/79, p. 1.
24 'Medicina rural y las brigadas internacionales', *MINSA Boletin Informativa 3*, 9/17/79, p. 1.
25 MINSA, *Logros y limitaciones en salud*, Managua: MINSA, 1980.
26 JGN, *La salud en Nicaragua antes y despues del de la revolucion*, Managua: MINSA, 1980.
27 Cruz JMC, 'La salud en la revolucion', *El Nuevo Diario*, 11/27/80, p. 4.
28 Echavarria F, 'Oficial Cubano de la salud publica habla de los problemas de salud', *Bohemia*, 2/8/80, pp. 60-63.
29 MINSA, *Reglamento general del servicio social rural*, Managua: MINSA, 1980.

Chapter 3

1 'The philosophies and policies of the Government of Nicaragua', In: Rosset P, Vandermeer J, eds, *The Nicaragua reader*, New York: Grove Press, 1983.
2 Kuhl CA, 'Mensaje del companero ministro de salud', *MINSA Boletin Informativa 1*, 9/7/79, p.3.
3 'Competitor or partner? Private practice in Nicaragua', *Nicaragua Health Fund Newsletter* 1989; 8: pp. 8-9.
4 For information on health care in Cost Rica see:
Antillon JJ, 'Changes in health care strategies in Costa Rica', *PAHO Bulletin* 1987; 21(2): 136-47.
Casas A, Vargas H, 'The health system in Costa Rica: toward a national health service', *Journal of Public Health Policy* 1980; 1:177-86.
Jaramillo J, Pineda C, Contreras G, 'Primary health care in marginal urban areas: the Costa Rican model', *PAHO Bulletin* 1984; 2:107-14.
Rosero-Bixby L, 'Las politicas socio-economicas y su efecto en el descenso de la mortalidad Costarricense', In: Associacion Demografico Costarricense, *Mortalidad y fecundidad en Costa Rica*, San Jose: ADC, 1984.
Rosero-Bixby L, 'Infant mortality decline in Costa Rica', In: Halstead SB, Walsh JA, Warren KS, eds, *Good health at low cost*, New York: Rockefeller Foundation, 1985.
Mohs E, 'Infectious diseases and health in Costa Rica: the development of a new paradigm', *Pediatric Infectious Disease* 1982; 3: 212-5.
Haines MR, Avery RC, 'Differential infant mortality in Costa Rica: 1968-1973', *Population Studies* 1982: 36(1): 31-44.
Gomes M, 'Servicos de saude para todos: o caso da Costa Rica', *Boletin de la Oficina Sanitaria Panamericana* 1986; 101(1): 58-73.
Saenz L, *Salud sin riqueza: el caso de Costa Rica*, San Jose: Ministerio de Salud, 1985.

5 For information on health care in Cuba see:
Stein Z, Susser M, 'The Cuban health system: a trial of a comprehensive service in a poor country', *International Journal of Health Services* 1972; 2(4): 551-66.
Danielson R, *Cuban medicine*, New Brunswick: Transaction Books, 1979.
Conover S, Donovan S, Susser E, 'Reflections of health care in Cuba', *The Lancet* 1980; 2: 958-60.
Navarro V, 'Health services in Cuba: an initial appraisal', *New England Journal of Medicine* 1972; 287: 954-9.
Ubell RN, 'High-tech medicine in the Caribbean: 25 years of Cuban health care', *New England Journal of Medicine* 1983; 309(23): 1468-72.
Muller F, Vila E, 'Participacion popular en la atencion sanitaria primaria en un area rural de Cuba, 1978', *Revista Cubana de Administracion de Salud* 1979; 5(3): 181-209.
Werner D, 'Health care in Cuba: a model service or a means of social control - or both?', In: Morley D, Rohde J, Williams G, *Practising health for all*, Oxford: Oxford University Press, 1983.
6 LeoGrande WM, 'The revolution in Nicaragua: another Cuba?', *Foreign Affairs* 1979; 58: 1.
7 Grant J, *State of the world's children report 1981/82*, New York: Oxford University Press, 1982.
see also: PAHO, *Child survival: priority health needs in Central America and Panama*, Washington, DC: PAHO, 1984.
Acuna HR, *Toward 2000: the quest for universal health in the Americas*, Washington DC: PAHO, 1983.
Acuna HR, 'Steps toward "Health for all by the year 2000": a review of PAHO's plan of action', *PAHO Bulletin* 1982; 16(1): 1-6.
8 WHO, *Declaration of Alma Ata: report on the international conference on primary health care*, Geneva: WHO, 1979.
9 Montis M, Molina G, Tercero I, Jarquin C, Jaramillo H, Bisso JM, Garcia N, Capote R, *Estrategias de atencion primaria de la salud en la republica de Nicaragua*, Managua: MIPLAN/MINSA, 1981.
10 Bohoslavsky A, 'La transformacion de la medicina en Nicaragua', *Barricada* 9/25/82, p. 3.
see also: 'Salud: metas y ojectivos para 1980', *Barricada* 12/24/79, p. 1.
11 Bossert TJ, 'Health care in revolutionary Nicaragua', In: Walker TW, ed, *Nicaragua in revolution*, New York: Praeger, 1982.
see also: Jones M, 'Nicaragua invests in health', *World Health* 1981; 12: 15-7.
12 Chamorro A, *Programa de extension de servicies de salud*, Managua: MINSA, 1980.
see also: MINSA, *Cartilla de salud para el alfabetizador*, Managua: MINSA, 1979.
'MINSA apoya la cruzada de alfabetizacion con 25 milliones de cordobas', *MINSA Boletin Informativa 8*, 1/29/80, p. 1.
13 Velasquez E, Hassan A, Belmar R, Drucker E, Michaels D, 'Occupational mercury poisoning in Nicaragua', *Morbidity and Mortality Weekly* 1980; 29(33): 393-95.
see also: Amador R, Lopez J, Garcia R, 'Research and development at the department of preventive medicine at the medical school of UNAN, Leon,

Nicaragua', *Scandinavian Journal of Social Medicine* 1988; 16: 235-6.
Aragon A, Pena R, Svanstrom L, Thorn A, 'Development of a community intervention programme on miners' health and working environment in Nicaragua', *Scandinavian Journal of Social Medicine* 1988; 16: 237-40.
14 Antonio Dager, unpublished manuscript.
15 MINSA, *El sistema nacional unico de salud: tres anos de revolucion 1979-1982*, Managua: MINSA, 1983.
16 Cuan M, Lopez MA, 'Evolucion y analysis de los servicios hospitalarios en Nicarauga', Masters' thesis, Managua: CIES, 1984.
17 'Salud va llegando poco a poco a todos los rincones', *El Nuevo Diario* 12/5/82, p. 4.
18 Eitel J, 'Health care revisited', *Nicaraguan Perspectives* 1986; 12: 30-6.
19 'Convenio INSS-MIDA-INRA: Centros de salud para unidades productivas', *El Nuevo Diario* 10/10/80, p. 9.
20 'Cada diez minutos una consulta medica', *Barricada* 3/3/82, p.1.
21 Miller V, *Between struggle and hope: the Nicaraguan literacy crusade*, Boulder: Westview Press, 1985.
22 MINSA, *Cartilla de malaria para los brigadistas de la campana de alfabetizacion*, Managua: MINSA, 1979.
23 'Escuela se convierte al instituto de salud', *Barricada* 7/4/80, p. 1.
24 Garfield RM, Taboada E, 'Health service reforms in revolutionary Nicaragua', *American Journal of Public Health* 1984: 74: 1138-44.
25 Lopez C, *Programa de extension de cobertura, regionalizacion, de los servicios de salud, segun region y area de salud*, Managua: MINSA, 1980.
26 MIPLAN, *Analisis del informe trimestral Enero-Marzo 1981*, Managua: MINSA, 1981.
27 Garfield RM, Taboada E, *op.cit.*
28 'Sorpresa: renuncia Amador', *La Prensa* 5/8/80, p. 1.

Chapter 4

1 Acuna HR, 'Community participation in the development of primary health services', *PAHO Bulletin* 1977; 9(2): 95-9.
see also: ECLAC, 'Popular participation in development', *Community Development Journal* 1973; 2: 77-92.
Gallardo LD, 'Algunas tendencias de la educacion y participacion comunitarias en salud en America Latina', *Boletin Oficial de la Organizacion Sanitaria Panamericana* 1984; 96(4): 314-24.
Muller F, *Participacion popular en programas de atencion sanitaria primaria en America Latina*, Medellin: Universidad de Antioquia, 1979.
Storms DM, *Training and use of auxiliary health workers: lessons from developing countries*, Washington DC: APHA International Health Programmes, 1979.
Stinson W, Favin M, Bradford B, *Training community health workers*, Washington: World Federation of Public Health Associations, 1983.
Hakim P, 'Lessons from grass-roots development experience in Latin America and the Carribbean', *Assignment Children* 1982; 59/60: 137-44.
WHO, *The community health worker*, Geneva: WHO, 1987.
2 Ministerio de Salud, *Politicas, estrategias y organizacion de la division de educacion para la salud*, Managua: Ministerio de Salud, 1975.

see also: USDHEW, *Syncrisis: the dynamics of health*, Publication No. (OS) 74-50007, Washington, DC: USGPO, 1978.
3 DECOPS, *Aportes para el analisis historico de la educacion y la participacion popular en salud*, Managua: MINSA, 1980.
see also: de Keyzer B, Ulate J, 'Educacion, participacion en salud e ideologia: Nicaragua pasado y presente', *Revista Centroamericana de Ciencias de la Salud* 1981; 17: 143-58.
4 Le Boterf G, 'The challenge of mass education in Nicaragua', *Assignment Children* 1984; 65/68: 247-66.
5 DECOPS, *Educacion y participacion comunitaria en la salud: lineamientos generales*, Managua: DECOPS, 1980.
6 DECOPS, 'Las jornadas populares: un proyecto de participacion popular en Nicaragua', *Revista Centramericano de Ciencias de la Salud* 1980: 17: 173-84.
7 DECOPS, *Manual operativo del capacitador, multiplicador, y brigadista popular de salud*, Managua: DECOPS, 1981.
8 Donahue JM, *The Nicaraguan revolution in health*, South Hadley: Bergin and Garvey, 1986.
9 Frieden T, Garfield R, 'Popular participation in health in Nicaragua', *Health Policy and Planning* 1987; 2(2): 162-70.
10 MINSA, *Objectivos, estructura, y funciones de la comision popular de salud*, Managua: MINSA, 1980.
11 'Primer consejo popular de salud del area 1 del centro de salud La Primavera', *MINSA Boletin Informativa 11*, 4/25/80, p. 1.
12 Comision de Salud de Leon, *Programa de capacitacion popular en salud*, Leon: Comision de Salud de Leon, 1979.
13 MINSA/Consejo Popular de Salud de Region 4, 'El papel de los consejos populares de salud en las jornadas populares de salud', *Primer Congreso Nacional JPS*, Managua: MINSA, 1984.
14 DECOPS, 'La educacion popular y las organizaciones de masas en la gestion de salud en Nicaragua', *Revista Centroamericano de Ciencias de la Salud* 1980; 17: 159-72.
15 Donahue JM, 'The politics of health care in Nicaragua before and after the revolution of 1979', *Human Organization* 1983; 42: 262-74.
16 Woznica C, 'Community participation in health as an empowering process: a case study from Nicaragua', DrPh Dissertation at University of Illinois at Chicago, 1987, p. 190.
17 *ibid.*, p. 189.
18 *ibid.*, p. 241.
19 *ibid.*, p. 196.
20 *ibid.*, p. 191.
21 *ibid.*, p. 192.
22 Garfield RM, Frieden T, 'Social and demographic characteristics of Nicaraguan health volunteers', *International Quarterly of Community Health Education* 1986-87; 7(2): 123-34.
23 MINSA, *La mujer Nicaraguense y su experiencia de participacion en salud*, Managua: MINSA, 1984.
24 Scholl EA, 'An assessment of community health workers in Nicaragua', *Social Science andd Medicine* 1985; 20: 207-14.

25 Ruchwarger G, *People in power: forging a grassroots democracy in Nicaragua*, South Hadley: Bergin and Garvey, 1987.
26 Cavallini I, 'Una critica sana', *Barricada Internacional* 9/8/88, p.14.
27 MINSA/Comision Popular de Salud Zona Especial II, 'Abriendo la trocha: brigadistas defienden salud y la revolucion en Zelaya Sur', *Primer Congreso Nacional JPS*, Managua: MINSA, 1984.
28 Rifkin SB, Muller F, Wolfgang B, 'Primary health care: on measuring participation', *Social Science and Medicine* 1988; 26(9): 931-40.
see also: Ugalde A, 'Ideological dimensions of community participation in Latin America health programmes', *Social Science and Medicine* 1985; 21(1): 41-53.
Kadt E, 'Community participation for health: the case of Latin America', *World Development* 1982; 10:573-84.
29 Woznica C, *op. cit.*, p. 258.
30 *ibid.*, p. 243.
31 *ibid.*, p. 244.
32 *ibid.* ,p. 281.
33 Shanks K, 'Poetry, puppets, and the people's health', *Nicaragua Health Fund Newsletter* 1988; 7: 7-9.
34 CIES, *La participacion popular como componente y estrategia de atencion primaria*, Managua: MINSA, 1983.

Chapter 5

1 Woznica C, 'Community participation in health as an empowering process: a case study from Nicaragua', DrPH Dissertation at University of Illinois at Chicago, 1987, pp. 218-219.
2 PAHO, 'Health conditions in the Americas', *Scientific Publication 364*, Washington, DC: PAHO, 1978.
3 de Castro JF, 'Mass vaccination against poliomyelitis in Mexico', *Review of Infectious Disease* 1984; 6(Supp.2): 397-99.
see also: Risi JB, 'The control of poliomyelitis in Brazil', *Review of Infectious Disease* 1984; 6(Supp 2): 404-12.
4 APHA, 'Nicaragua: 40,000 health volunteers vaccinate a nation', *Salubritas* 1981; 5(3): 1-2.
see also: MINSA, *Plan nacional de medicina preventiva*, Managua: MINSA, 1980.
5 Estimates from MINSA, as reported to PAHO and published in PAHO, 'Health conditions in the Americas 1977-1980', *Scientific Publication 427*, Washington, DC: PAHO, 1982.
6 Williams G, 'Immunisation in Nicaragua', *The Lancet* 1985; 15(4): 780.
7 Estimates from MINSA, as reported to PAHO and published in PAHO: *op. cit.*
8 Wernsdorfer WH, 'The Importance of malaria in the world', In: Kreier JP, ed, *Malaria, Volume one: epidemiology, chemotherapy, morphology, and metabolism*, New York: Academic Press, 1980.
see also: Harrison G, *Mosquitoes, malaria, and man*, New York: Dutton, 1978.
9 'Sera como la alfabetizacion: cruzada anti-malarica', *El Nuevo Diario* 9/19/81, p. 1.

10 Garfield RM, Vermund SH, 'Health education and community participation in mass drug administration for malaria in Nicaragua', *Social Science and Medicine* 1986; 22(8): 869-77.
11 'Medicos ofrecen ayuda en plan anti-malarico', *La Prensa* 10/23/81, p.6.
12 Garfield RM, Vermund SH, 'Changes in malaria incidence after a mass drug administration in Nicaragua', *The Lancet* 1983; 2: 500-3.
see also: Garfield RM, Vermund SH, 'Malaria in Nicaragua: an update', *The Lancet* 1984; 1: 1125.
Bruce-Chwatt LJ, 'Mass drug administration for control of malaria', *The Lancet* 1983; 2: 688.
Foll C, 'Mass drug administration for control of malaria', *The Lancet* 1983; 2: 1022.
13 PAHO, *Status of malaria control programmes in the Americas: 36th annual report*, Washington, DC: PAHO, 1988.
14 Garfield RM, Prado E, Gates JR, Vermund SH, 'Malaria in Nicaragua: community-based control efforts and the impact of war', *International Journal of Epidemiology* 1989; 18(2).
see also: Sweezey SI, Murray DL, Dax RG, 'Nicaragua's revolution in pesticide policy', *Environment* 1986; 28(1): 6-36.
15 Loevinsohn BP, Loevinsohn ME, 'Well-child clinics and mass vaccination campaigns: an evaluation of strategies for improving the coverage of primary health care in a developing country', *American Journal of Public Health* 1987; 77(11): 1407-11.

Chapter 6

1 JGN, *Contrarrevolucion: dessarrollo y conscuencias, datos basicos, 1980 - 1985*, JGN: Managua, 1985.
see also: INSSBI, *48 meses de aggression extranjera*, Managua: INSSBI, 1984.
Perez B, 'Efectos epidemiologicos de la guerra de aggression', Presentation at the 3rd Annual US-Nicaragua Health Colloquium, Managua, November 1985.
CAHI, 'Nicaragua 1984: human and material costs of the war', In: Rosset P, Vandermeer J, *Nicaragua: unfinished revolution*, New York: Grove Press, 1986.
Kornbluh P, *Nicaragua, the price of intervention: Reagan's war against the Sandinistas*, Washington DC: Institute for Policy Studies, 1987.
Garfield RM, 'Health and the war against Nicaragua, 1981-1984', *Journal of Public Health Policy* 1985; 6(1): 116-31.
Garfield RM, Frieden T, Vermund SH, 'Health related outcomes of war in Nicaragua', *American Journal of Public Health* 1987; 77(5): 615-8.
Siegel D, Baron R, Epstein P, 'The epidemiology of aggression', *The Lancet* 1985; 1: 1492-3.
Garfield R, 'Health consequences of war in Nicaragua', *The Lancet* 1985; 2: 392.
2 INEC, *Efectos socio-economicos de la guerra de agresion*, Managua: INEC, 1988.
3 Personal communication, Tim Takaro and MINSA workers in Region 6.
4 INEC, *op. cit.*
see also: INSSBI, *Repercusion del terrorismo de estado de la administracion*

Reagan en la vida del pueblo Nicaraguense, Managua: Comite Nacional de Emergencia, 1984.
Kinzer S, 'Casualties in Nicaragua: schools and health care', *New York Times* 3/23/87, p. 10.
5 MINSA, *Plan de salud 1988-90*, Managua: MINSA, 1987.
6 JGN, *Contrarrevolucion: dessarrollo y conscuencias, datos basicos, 1980 - 1985*, Managua: JGN, 1985.
see also: MINSA, 'Repercusion de la agresion en la situacion de salud del pais', *El Nuevo Diario* 8/9/83, p.13.
7 Almasi MS, *Desarrollo del sector farmaeutico de Nicaragua*, Geneva: United Nations Industrial Development Organization, 1985.
8 Leahy S, 'Captured by the contra', *Nicaragua Health Fund Newsletter* 1987; 2: 3-5.
9 'The philosophies and policies of the government of Nicaragua', In: Rosset P, Vandermeer J, eds, *The Nicaragua reader*, New York: Grove Press, 1983.
10 Garfield RM, 'War-related changes in health and health services in Nicaragua', *Social Science and Medicine* 1989; 28(7): 669-76.
see also: Sivard RL, *World military and social expenditures 1985*, Washington, DC: Worldwatch Institute, 1985.
11 MINSA, *Plan de salud 1987*, Managua: MINSA, 1986.
12 Kinzer S, 'Land mines in Nicaragua cause rising casualties', *New York Times* 7/19/86, p.5.
13 Gogstad A, 'Rehabilitation in war-ravaged developing countries', *Rehabilitation Literature* 1978; 38: 5-8.
14 Garfield RM. *op. cit.*
15 MINSA/Comision Popular de Salud Zona Especial II, 'Abriendo la trocha: brigadistas defienden salud y la revolucion en Zelaya Sur', *Primer Congreso Nacional JPS*, Managua: MINSA, 1984.
16 Meyer H, 'Physician's war in Nicaragua', *American Medical News* 11/13/87, p. 3.
17 CAHI, 'The other side of the border: Nicaragua's internal refugees', *CAHI Update* 1985; 14: 1-4.
18 Garfield RM, Prado E, Gates JR, Vermund SH, 'Malaria in Nicaragua: community-based control efforts and the impact of war', *International Journal of Epidemiology* 1989; 18(2).
19 On related topics see:
Dudley HAF, Knight RJ, McNeur JC, Rosengarten DS, 'Civilian battle casualties in Vietnam', *British Journal of Surgery* 1968; 55: 332.
see also: Hartigan RS, *The forgotten victim: a history of the civilian*, Chicago: Precedent Publishing, Inc., 1982.
20 'Barcos yanquis bloquean medicinas para el pueblo', *El Nuevo Diario* 10/7/83, p. 1.
21 Humphries SV, 'The mental effects of guerrilla warfare', *Central African Journal of Medicine* 1978; 24: 37-39.
see also: Summerfield D, 'Nicaragua: war and mental health', *The Lancet* 1987; 2:914.
Summerfield D, 'The psychological war', *Nicaragua Health Fund Newsletter* 1987; 2: 3-5.
Whitford JD, 'Consecuencias psicologicas derivadas de la situacion de

guerra', *Psicologia en Nicaragua* 1987; 1(1): 10-15.
22 CARE, *Children's survival assistance programme. Needs assessment team field report: Nicaragua*, New York: CARE, 1988.
see also: Nelson H, 'War takes toll on children in Nicaragua', *American Medical News* 2/17/89, p. 3.
23 INEC, *Efectos socio-economicos de la guerra de agresion,* Managua: INEC,1988.
24 Cliff J, Noormahomed AR, 'Health as a target: South Africa's destabilization of Mozambique', *Social Science and Medicine* 1988; 27(7): 717-22. .
25 Walt G, Melamed A, eds, *Mozambique: towards a people's health service*, London: Zed Press, 1984.
26 Waghelstein JW, 'Post-Vietnam counterinsurgency doctrine', *Military Review* 1985; 1: 42.
27 Kornbluh P, *Nicaragua, the price of intervention: Reagan's war against the Sandinistas*, Washington DC: Institute for Policy Studies, 1987.
28 Keegan J, *The face of battle*, New York: Penguin, 1976.
29 Kornbluh P, *op. cit.*
30 Braveman P, Siegel D, 'Nicaragua: a health system developing under conditions of war', *International Journal of Health Service* 1987; 17: 169-78.
31 'Plan de atencion medica antes un eventual invasion', *Barricada* 11/22/84, p.12.
32 Jackson S, 'How to bring health care to war zone communities', *Nicaragua Health Fund Newsletter* 1988; 8:4-7.
33 'The challenge of health care in the Nicaraguan countryside', *CEPAD Report* 1989; 1: 1-4.
34 Schneider ML, 'Health as a bridge for peace', *World Health* 1987; 10: 5-6.

Chapter 7

1 Ortega D, *Daniel y los medicos de Nicaragua: problemas, medidas y compromiso*, Managua: Direccion de Informacion y Prensa de la Presidencia de la Republica, 1985.
2 Tamayo JO, 'Public health system is ailing in Nicaragua', *The Miami Herald* 11/30/85, p. 1.
3 UNICEF, *Datos basicos e indicadores economicos, humanos, politicos, y sociales sobre Nicaragua*, Managua: UNICEF, 1988.
see also: Gariazzo A, Acosta M, Bermudez A, *Analisis de la situacion economico-social de Nicaragua*, Managua: UNICEF, 1984.
4 Braveman P, 'Primary health care takes root in Nicaragua', *World Health Forum* 1985; 6: 369-72.
5 Bossert T, 'Nicaraguan health policy: the dilemma of success', *Medical Anthropology Quarterly* 1984; 15(3): 73-4.
see also: Bosche MA, *Development of primary health care in Nicaragua: achievements and difficulties*, Managua: MINSA, 1983.
MIPLAN/MINSA, *Estrategias de atencion primaria de la salud en la Republica de Nicaragua*, Managua: MIPLAN y MINSA, 1981.
6 MINSA, *Guia de programacion de actividades para el desarrollo de la estrategia de atencion primaria a nivel de region y area de salud*, Managua: MINSA, 1983.
7 MINSA, *Plan integral de actividades del area de salud - libro rojo y negro*,

Managua: MINSA, 1982.
8 MINSA, *Plan de salud 1987*, Managua: MINSA, 1986.
9 Slater RG, 'Reflections on curative health care in Nicaragua', *American Journal of Public Health* 1989; 79(5): 646-51.
10 Ortega D, *op. cit.*
11 'Lea Guido: hay sectores inmaduros e incomprensivos', *El Nuevo Diario* 8/7/81, p. 6.
12 'Comentan nombramiento en salud', *La Prensa* 7/2/85, p. 1.
13 Wilson PA, 'Regionalization and decentralization in Nicaragua', *Latin American Perspectives* 1987; 14(2): 237-54.
14 OMS/OPS/UNICEF, *Documentos basicos de coordinacion de la cooperacion interagencial en Nicaragua*, Managua: OPS/UNICEF, 1985.
15 Werner D, *Donde no hay doctor: una guia para los campesinos que viven lejos de los centros medicos*, Palo Alto: La Fundacion Hesperian, 1980.
16 MINSA, *Plan de salud 1987*, Managua: MINSA, 1986.
17 'A survival economy', *Envio* 1985; 4: 52.
18 Borsari A, Sessa C, Flores B, *Proyecto de un programa piloto de deteccion del cancer del cuello uterino en el area de salud no. 6 region III*, Managua: MINSA, 1987.
19 'A survival economy', *Envio* 1985; 4: 52.
20 *ibid.*
21 Escudero JC, 'Los sistemas de informacion en salud en America Latina', *Revista Centroamericano de Ciencias de la Salud* 1979; 14: 109-22.
22 Palloni A, 'Mortality in Latin America: emerging patterns', *Population Development Review* 1981; 7(4): 623-49.
see also: Monto AS, Johnson KM, 'Respiratory infections in the American tropics', *American Journal of Tropical Medicine and Hygiene* 1968; 17(8): 867-71.
Delgado HL, Giron EM, de Leon H, Hurtado E, 'Epidemiology of acute respiratory infection in preschool children of rural Guatemala', *PAHO Bulletin* 1988: 22(4); 383-93.
23 Oficina de Vigilancia Epidemiologica, 'Evaluacion de la vigilancia epidemiologica primer trimestre 1987', *Boletin Epidemiologico Nicaraguense* 1987; 2: 1-3.
see also: Cole DC, McConnell R, Murry DL, Anton FP, 'Pesticide illness surveillance: the Nicaraguan experience', *PAHO Bulletin* 1988; 22(2): 119-32.
24 MINSA, 'Analisis de la vigilancia epidemiologica del ano 1986', *Boletin Epidemiologico Nicaraguense* 1987; 1: 1-3.
25 Wilson PA, *op. cit.*
26 MINSA, Region 3, *Algunas ideas sobre el medico del barrio*, Managua: MINSA, 1989.
27 Danielson R, *Cuban medicine*, New Brunswick: Transaction Books, 1979.

Chapter 8

1 Deighton J, Horsley R, Stewart S, Cain C, *Sweet ramparts: women in revolutionary Nicaragua*, London: War on Want, 1983.
2 MINSA, *Normas de atencion prenatal*, Managua: MINSA, 1984.
3 MINSA, *Plan de salud 1986,* Managua: MINSA, 1985.
4 MINSA, *Plan de salud 1988-90*, Managua: MINSA, 1987.

5 MINSA, *Plan de salud 1988-90*, Managua: MINSA, 1987.
6 Houtart F, Lemercinier G, *Creencias y practicas que conciernen a la salud, en los grupos populares rurales y urbanos Nicaraguense*, Louvain-la-Neuve: Universite Catholique de Louvain, 1984.
7 Norory M, 'Abortion in Nicaragua', *Nicaragua Health Fund Newsletter* 1987; 4: 7.
8 PAHO, *Health of women in the Americas*, Washington, DC: PAHO, 1985. *see also*: WHO, *Maternal mortality rates*, Geneva: WHO Bulletin 1985; 2.
9 MINSA, *Plan de salud 1988-90*, Managua: MINSA, 1987. *see also*: Guido C, Garcia M, Navas D, 'Analisis de 2746 abortos atendidos en el hospital general de Nicaragua', *International Surgery* 1971; 56(2): 125-7.
10 Altamirano L, 'Aborto inducido ilegalmente: costos y consequencias', Presentation at Jornada Cientifica Nacional de Salud, Managua, 11/85.
11 ADN, *Resultados de la encuesta sobre conocimiento, actitud, y practica hacia la educacion sexual y planificacion familiar*, Managua: ADN, 1978.
12 Lebrun JF, *La imagen de los centros de salud en los medios populares de Nicaragua*, Louvain-la-Neuve: Centro Tricontinental, 1984.
13 Heiby JR, 'Low-cost health delivery systems: lessons from Nicaragua', *American Journal of Public Health* 1981; 71(5): 514-9.
14 Norory M, *op. cit.*
15 Luisier V, *Te voy a ayudar nada mas...apuntes sobre las parteras empiricas en Nicaragua*, Managua: MINS, 1985.
16 Colectiva del libro de salud de las mujeres de Boston, *Nuestros cuerpos, nuestras vidas: un libro por y para las mujeres*, Boston: The Boston Women's Health Book Collective, 1979.
17 Borge T, 'Women's liberation in Nicaragua', Speech in Leon, Nicaragua, 9/29/82. Translated and published in *Intercontinental Press* 11/1/82, pp. 794-800.
18 'Planning health care for women', *Nicaragua Health Fund Newsletter* 1987; 4: 6-7.

Chapter 9

1 Miller V, *Between struggle and hope: the Nicaraguan literacy crusade*, Boulder: Westview Press, 1985.
2 CIERA/PAN/CIDA, *Informe del primer seminario sobre estrategia alimentaria*, Managua: CIERA, 1983.
3 MINSA, *El sistema nacional unico de salud: tres anos de revolucion 1979-1982*, Managua: MINSA, 1983.
4 CELADE, *La mortalidad en la ninez en Centroamerican, Panama and Belice: Nicaragua 1970-1986*, San Jose: CELADE, 1988.
5 Silva F, *La salud del nino*, Managua: Ministerio de Cultura, 1986.
6 Terra JP, 'The major problems affecting children in Latin America', *Assignment Children* 1979; 47/48: 79-91. *see also*: Puffer RR, Serrano CV, 'Patterns of mortality in childhood', *Scientific Publication 262*, Washington, DC: PAHO, 1973. Grosse RN, 'Interrelation between health and population: observations derived from field experiences', *Social Science and Medicine* 1980; 14c: 99-120.

Baum S, Arriaga E, 'Levels, trends, differentials, and causes of early childhood mortality in Latin America', *World Health Statistics Quarterly* 1981; 34(3): 147-67.
Behm H, 'Mortalidad en los primeros anos de vida en paises de America Latina', *CELADE, Serie A, 1024-1032 y 1036-1039*, Costa Rica: CELADE, 1976-78.
Behm H, 'Mortalidad en America Central: realidad actual y perspectivas', *Revista Centroamericana de Ciencias de Salud* 1981; 9: 9-35.
7 MINSA, *Programa control de enfermedades diarreicas*, Managua: MINSA, 1980.
see also: Scardino PT, 'Bacterial diarrhoea in eastern Nicaragua', *Southern Medical Journal* 1971; 64(7): 823-9.
Zeldin L, *El impacto de la terapia de rehidratacion oral en Nicaragua y perspectivas*, Managua: MINSA/CIES, 1985.
8 Heiby JR, 'Low-cost health delivery systems: lessons from Nicaragua', *American Journal of Public Health* 1981; 71: 514-9.
9 Hirschhorn N, 'Oral rehydration therapy: the programme and the promise', In: Cash R, Keusch GT, Lamstein J, *Child health and survival*, Helm: Wolfboro, 1987.
10 MINSA, 'Diarrhoeal diseases control programme', *Weekly Epidemiology Record* 1985; 60: 93-100.
11 Garfield RM, Siu C, Arguello CA, Frieden T, Vermund SH, Williams G, 'Impact of diarrhoea control programmes in Nicaragua, 1980-1986', unpublished.
12 MINSA, 'Diarrhoeal diseases control programme', *Weekly Epidemiology Record* 1985; 60: 93-100.
13 Sequeira M, Valdez L, 'Estudio clinico epidemiologic de fallecidos menores de 5 anos por enfermedad diarreica aguada en Region III, 1985', *Boletin Epidemiologico Nicaraguense* 1987; 1:10-11.
see also: Torres OD, 'Determinantes de la morbi-mortalidad por enfermedad diarreica de los menores de cinco anos que acuden a los hospitales infantiles de Managua', Master's thesis. Managua: CIES, 1986.
14 MINSA, *Manejo de la enfermedad diarreica aguda y la deshidratacion segun nivel de atencion*, Managua: MINSA, 1985.
15 MINSA. *Plan de salud 1988-1990*, Managua: MINSA, 1987.
16 Watson G, 'Desarrollo y perspectivas del programa atencion materno infantil', *Boletin Nicaraguense de Higiene y Epidemiologia* 1984; 1(2): 33-43.
17 Interview with Dr. Fernando Silva, *Barricada Internacional* 9/8/88, p. 4.
18 Ministerio de Salud, *Sumario de estudios sobre el estatado nutricional de la poblacion*, Managua: Ministerio de Salud, 1974.
19 Unpublished data generated by a study reported in Wolfe BL, Behrman I, 'Determinants of child mortality, health, and nutrition in a developing country', *Journal of Development Economics* 1982; 11: 163-93.
20 Lindenburg C, *Estudio sobre los effectos del acercamiento temprano madre-infante sobre la incidencia y duracion de la lactancia materna*, Managua: MINSA, 1983.
21 MINSA, *Primer taller nacional sobre lactancia materna*, Managua: MINSA, 1980.
see also: Area Materno-infantil, *Programa de lactancia materna*, Managua:

MINSA, 1981.
22 O'Leary de Macias G, 'A women's movement in Nicaragua, an advocate of breast-feeding', *Assignment Children* 1981: 55/56: 117-30.
23 MINSA/CIES, *Enfoque de riesgo y estado nutricional de los ninos menores de 5 anos en la region 3*, Managua: CIES, 1988.
24 Tefel RA, Mendoza H, Flores J, 'Social welfare', In: Walker T, ed, *Nicaragua: The first five years*, New York: Praeger, 1985.
25 MINSA/CIES, *Enfoque de riesgo y estado nutricional de los ninos menores de 5 anos en la region 3*, Managua: CIES, 1988.
26 Trowbridge FL, Newton LH, 'Seasonal changes in malnutrition and diarrhoeal disease among preschool children in El Salvador', *American Journal of Tropical Medicine and Hygiene* 1979; 28(1): 136-41.
see also: Teller C, Sibrian R, Talavera C, Bent V, Del Canto J, Saenz L, 'Population and nutrition: implications of sociodemographic trends and differentials for food and nutrition policy in Central America and Panama', *Ecology of Food and Nutrition* 1979; 8: 95-109.
Teller CH, 'Demografia de la desnutricion en America Central', *Intercom* 1981: 6-9.
May JM, McLellan DL, 'The republic of Nicaragua', In: May JM, McLellan DL, *The ecology of malnutrition in Mexico and Central America*, New York: Hafner, 1972.
Delgado HL, Valverde V. Belizan JM, Klein RE, 'Diarrhoeal diseases, nutritional status and health care: analysis of their interrelationships', *Ecology, Food and Nutrition* 1983; 12: 229-34.
27 Aburto A, *Primer censo nacional de talla en escolares de primer grado de primaria de la Republica de Nicaragua*, Managua: PAN, 1986.
see also: Palacios MA, Romero A, 'Situacion y perspectiva de la nutricion en Nicaragua', *Boletin Nicaraguense de Higiene y Epidemiologia* 1984; 1(1): 55-8.
28 CARE, *Children's survival assistance programme. Needs assessment team field report: Nicaragua*, New York: CARE, 1988.
29 INEC, *Efectos socio-economicos de la guerra de agresion*, Managua: INEC, 1988.
30 CELADE, *La mortalidad en la ninez en Centroamerican, Panama and Belice: Nicaragua 1970-1986*, San Jose: CELADE, 1988.
31 UNICEF, *Datos basicos e indicadores economicos, humanos, politicos, y sociales sobre Nicaragua*, Managua: UNICEF, 1988.
32 CELADE, *La mortalidad en la ninez en Centroamerican, Panama and Belice: Nicaragua 1970-1986*, San Jose: CELADE, 1988.
33 Morales E, Oporta R, et al, *La sobrevivencia de ninos en Nicaragua: resultados preliminares de estudios en 33 sitios sentinelas sobre la mortalidad infantil en las regiones II, III, y V*, Managua: MINSA, 1988.
34 CELADE, *La mortalidad en la ninez en Centroamerican, Panama y Belice: caracteristicas principales*, San Jose: CELADE, 1988.
35 CELADE, *La mortalidad en la ninez en Centroamerican, Panama and Belice: Nicaragua 1970-1986*, San Jose: CELADE, 1988.
36 'El drama de la salud infantil', *Pensamento Proprio* 1988; 6: 44-8.
37 Cerezo LV, Rodriguez A, Duran R, *Frecuencia de factores de alto riesgo obstetrico*, Managua: MINSA, 1983.

see also: Hernandez B, Jimenez V, 'Enfoque de riesgo: estrategia para la atencion primaria en Nicaragua', *Salud y Ciencia en la Revolucion* 1984; 1(1): 19-21.
MINSA/CIES, *Enfoque de riesgo y estado nutricional de los ninos menores de 5 anos en la region 3*, Managua: CIES, 1988.
38 Behm H, 'Socio-economic determinants of mortality in Latin America', *Population Bulletin of the United Nations* 1980; 13: 1-15.
see also: Carvajal M, Burgess P, 'Socioeconomic determinants of foetal and child deaths in Latin America', *Social Science and Medicine* 1978: 12(C): 89-98.
Scrimshaw SCM, Hurtado E, 'Anthropological involvement in the Central American diarrhoeal disease control project', *Social Science and Medicine* 1988; 27(1): 97-105.
Mata L, 'Diarrhoeal disease - how Costa Rica won', *World Health Forum* 1981; 1: 141-45.
Mata L, 'The evolution of diarrhoeal disease and malnutrition in Costa Rica', *Assignment Children* 1983; 61/62: 195-224.

Chapter 10
1 Danielson R, *Cuban medicine*, New Brunswick: Transaction Books, 1979.
2 Belmar R, Sidel VW, 'An international perspective on strikes and threatened strikes by physicians', *International Journal of Health Services* 1975; 5(27): 53.
3 As many as 50 Nicaraguans trained as physicians in the Soviet Union during the 1970s. While most of them returned to Nicaragua following the Sandinista revolution, they seem to have followed no particular political trend. Like other Nicaraguan physicians, few are FSLN members. Most have private practices, and many have emigrated.
4 'Proyecto regulador preocupa a medicos', *La Prensa* 8/18/80, p. 5.
5 'La medicina como comercio', *El Nuevo Diario* 12/12/84, p. 2.
6 The precise number of physicians who have emigrated is not known. This estimate was made by the professional association, CONAPRO, based on information from MINSA and the Ministry of the Interior.
7 'Politica de estimulos a la profesion medica', *El Nuevo Diario* 6/10/85, p. 2.
8 'Proyecto regulador preocupa a medicos', *La Prensa* 8/18/80, p. 5.
9 Garfield RM, Taboada E, 'Health service reforms in revolutionary Nicaragua', *American Journal of Public Health* 1984: 74: 1138-44.
10 'Por que se van los doctores', *La Prensa* 6/12/85, p. 2.
11 'Medicos con multiples quejas', *El Nuevo Diario* 6/23/85, p. 1.
12 'Competitor or partner? Private practice in Nicaragua', *Nicaragua Health Fund Newsletter* 1989; 8: 8-9.
13 'Normaran la actividad de la medicina privada', *Barricada* 12/24/88, p.1.
14 Alvarez E, 'Medicina privada: eficiente y economica', *La Prensa* 1/5/89, p.3.
15 Braveman PA, Roemer, MI, 'Health personnel training in the Nicaraguan health system', *International Journal of Health Services* 1985; 15(4): 699-705.
16 Haddad J, 'Estado actual de la ensenanza de la salud publica en Centroamerica y Panama', *Educacion Medica y Salud* 1982; 16(11): 69-76.
see also: Morley D, 'Medical education in the developing world - new

approaches needed', *Medical Teacher* 1979; 1(5): 258-61.
17 Facultad de Ciencias Medicas, *La educacion medica en Nicaragua: situacion actual, logros y perspectivas*, Managua: UNAN, 1981.
18 '25 estudiantes de medicina hacia las zonas combate', *Barricada* 6/1/84, p.10.
19 Perez R, *La formacion de personal especializado en salud publica: experiencia de Nicaragua*, Managua: MINSA, 1984.
20 Galiano S, 'Brief history of nursing in Nicaragua', *International Journal of Nursing Studies* 1975; 12: 223-9.
21 de Borge Z, Malespin C, Herrera de Tercero N, Pineda A, *Perfil profesional de la enfermera y su responsibilidad ante la sociedad actual*, Managua: Colegio de Enfermeras Nicaraguenses, 1980.
22 Garfield RM, 'Health in Nicaragua today: interview with Concepcion Huerte Ramirez', *Catalyst* 1980; 2(4): 45-54.
23 Molina G, *Situacion actual y perspectiva de desarrollo en la carrera de enfermeria a nivel tecnico y superior*, Managua: MINSA, 1985.
24 Garfield RM, 'The evolution of nursing in Nicaragua', *Nursing Outlook* 1988; 36(1): 25-9.
25 Lewis C, Squires A, 'Where every plaster counts: the reality of nursing in Nicaragua', *Nicaragua Health Fund Newsletter* 1988; 6: 1-2.
26 'Descentralizar la formacion de especialists medicos, tecnicos, y las enfermeras', *Barricada* 2/15/84, p. 7.
27 Ugalde A, 'Where there is a doctor: strategies to increase productivity at lower costs', *Social Science and Medicine* 1984; 19(4): 441-50.

Chapter 11

1 Houtart F, Lemercinier G, *Creencias y practicas que conciernen a la salud, en los grupos populares rurales y urbanos Nicaraguense*, Louvain-la-Neuve: Universite Catholique de Louvain, 1984.
2 'Como acabar con anarquia y explotacion con medicinas', *El Nuevo Diario* 8/21/81, p. 1.
3 For a discussion of the tuberculosis situation, see:
'Taking on TB', *Nicaragua Health Fund Newsletter* 1987; 4: 1- 3.
MINSA, *Informe sobre la situacion de la tuberculosis en Nicaragua*, Managua: MINSA, 1980.
4 MINSA, *Plan de salud 1988-1990*, Managua: MINSA, 1987.
5 Cortes G, 'A parar la guerra de las hormigas', *Barricada* 4/21/82, p.4.
6 Hernandez L, 'Al "reventar" inventarios de medicamentos', *Barricada* 8/25/88, p.1.
7 Ruiz M, Sanchez R, 'Medicamentos como insumos criticos', Masters' thesis, Managua: CIES, 1984.
8 CAM, *La producion e importacion de medicamentos y la problematica de la Central de Abastecimientos Medicos*, Managua: MINSA, 1981.
9 PAHO, 'Essential drugs revolving fund for Central America and Panama', *PAHO Bulletin* 1988; 22(3): 313-6.
see also: Laporte J, Tognoni G, 'Drug policy in Nicaragua', *Development Dialogue* 1985; 2: 121-8.
10 MINSA, *Formulario nacional de medicamentos*, Managua: MINSA, 1985.
11 Almasi MS, *Desarrollo del sector farmaeutico de Nicaragua*, Geneva: United Nations Industrial Development Organization, 1985.

12 'A survival economy', *Envio* 1985; 4: 52.
13 Green D, 'Rescuing their roots: herbal medicine', *Nicaragua Health Fund Newsletter* 1987; 3: 5-6.
14 Sotomayor U, Cardoza J, Brussel J, 'Rescate de la medicina popular en el uso, aplicacion y cultivo de plantas medicinales en Region I', *Salud* 1987; 1(1): 40-43.
15 But this is a profoundly complex issue. See:
Bonair A, Rosenfield P, Tengyald K, 'Medical technologies in developing countries: issues of technology development, transfer, diffusion, and use', *Social Science and Medicine* 1989; 28(8): 769-81.
Joseph SC, 'Iron axe, magic lamp, or Trojan horse: issues in cross-cultural transfer of health technology', In: James G, Sax Jacoles B, *The technology explosion in medical science: implications for the health care industry and the public*, New York: SP Medical and Scientific Books, 1983.
16 MINSA, *Plan de salud 1988-1990*, Managua: MINSA, 1987.
17 Mitchell EL, Martinez-Silva R, Vardham H, Vazques IA, 'Administracion, mantenimiento y reparacion de equipos para laboratorios en los paises en desarrollo', *Boletin de la Organizacion Sanitaria Panamericana* 1983; 95(5):393-408.
18 MINSA, *Plan de salud 1988-1990*, Managua: MINSA, 1987.

Chapter 12

1 Zschock DK, *Health care financing in developing countries*, Washington DC: APHA, 1979.
see also: Gish O, Feller LL, *Planning pharmaceuticals for primary health care*, Washington DC: APHA, 1979.
2 Zschock DK, *op. cit.*
3 PAHO, *National and international financial and budgeting implications of regional strategies and the plan of action for health for all by the year 2000*, Washington DC: PAHO, WHO, 1984.
4 OMS/OPS/UNICEF, *Documentos basicos de coordinacion de la cooperacion interagencial en Nicaragua*, Managua: OPS/UNICEF, 1986.
5 MINSA, *Health plan 1988-1990*, Managua: MINSA, 1987.
6 INEC, *Efectos socio-economicos de la guerra de agresion*, Managua: INEC, 1988.

Chapter 13

1 ECLA, *Nicaragua: Economic repercussions of recent political events*, Santiago de Chile: United Nations, 1979
2 Fagen R, Deere CD, Coraggio JL, eds, *Transition and development: problems of third world socialism*, New York: Monthly Review Press, 1986.
see also: 'The philosophies and policies of the government of Nicaragua', In: Rosset P, Vandermeer J, eds, *The Nicaragua reader*, New York: Grove Press, 1983.
Vilas CM, *Perfiles de la revolucion Sandinista*, Buenos Aires: Editorial Legasa, 1984.
3 Walker TW, ed, *Reagan versus the Sandinistas*, Boulder: Westview Press, 1987.
4 Miller V, *Between struggle and hope: the Nicaraguan literacy crusade*,

Boulder: Westview Press, 1985.
see also: Le Boterf G, 'The challenge of mass education in Nicaragua', *Assignment Children* 1984; 65/68: 247-66.
5 Tefel RA, Mendoza H, Flores J, 'Social welfare', In: Walker T, ed, *Nicaragua: The first five years*, New York: Praeger, 1985.
6 UNICEF, *Datos basicos e indicadores economicos, humanos, politicos, y sociales sobre Nicaragua*, Managua: UNICEF, 1988.
7 Gariazzo A, Acosta M, Bermudez A, *Analisis de la situacion economico-social de Nicaragua*, Managua: UNICEF, 1984.
8 *ibid.*
9 *ibid.*
10 CIERA/ATC/UNAG, *Produccion y organizacion en el agro Nicaraguense*, Managua: CIERA, 1982.
11 UNICEF, *op. cit.*
12 *ibid.*
13 Barraclough SL, Scott MF, *The rich have already eaten*, Amsterdam: Transnational Institute, 1987.
14 Ministerio de Salud, *Diagnostico del sector salud de Nicaragua*, Managua: Ministerio de Salud, 1975.
15 Collins J, *et al*, *Nicaragua: what difference could a revolution make?*, New York: Grove Press, 1986.
16 Zalkin M, 'Food policy and class transformation in revolutionary Nicaragua, 1979 - 1986', *World Development* 1987; 15(7): 961-84.
17 *ibid.*
18 *ibid.*
19 Collins J *et al*, *op. cit.*
20 Barraclough SL, Scott MF, *op. cit.*
21 Fitzgerald V, 'Agrarian reform as a model of accumulation: the case of Nicaragua since 1979', *Journal of Development Studies* 1985; 22(1).
22 Zalkin M, *op. cit*
23 CEPAL, *Istmo Centroamericano: crisis economica y planificacion del desarrollo*, LC/MEX/R.2, Mexico: CEPAL, 1985.
see also: Musgrove P, 'The economic crisis and its impact on health and health care in Latin America and the Caribbean', *International Journal of Health Services* 1987; 17(3): 411.
Musgrove P, 'Impact of the economic crisis on health and health care in Latin America and the Caribbean', *WHO Chronicles* 1986; 40(4): 152-7.
24 'A survival economy', *Envio* 1985; 4: 52.
25 Zalkin M, *op. cit.*
26 Barraclough SL, Scott MF, *op. cit.*
27 Austin J, Fox J, Kruger W, 'The role of the revolutionary state in the Nicaraguan food system', *World Development* 1985; 13(1): 15-40.
28 *Barricada Internacional* 1988; 34: 261: p. 10.
29 Uhlig MA, 'Nicaraguan study depicts economy in drastic decline', *New York Times* 1/26/89, p. 1.
30 MINSA, *Health plan 1987*, Managua: MINSA, 1986.
31 'How will Nicaragua survive hurricane Joan?', *Nicaragua Health Fund Newsletter* 1989; 9: 1-4.
see also: ECLAC, *Report on damage caused to Nicaragua by hurricane Joan*,

New York: United Nations, 1988.

Chapter 14

1 Bommer J, 'The politics of disaster - Nicaragua', *Disasters* 1985; 9(4): 270-8.
2 See the tables in Grant J, *State of the world's children report, 1989*, London: Oxford University Press, 1988.
3 Zukin P, 'Health and economic development: how significant is the relationship?', *International Development Review* 1975; 2: 17-21.
see also: Chen LC, 'Coping with economic crisis: policy development in China and India', *Health Policy and Planning* 1987; 2(2): 138-49.
Bell D, Reich M, eds, *Health, nutrition, and economic crises*, Dover, Mass: Auburn House, 1986.
4 Coraggio JL, Deere CD, eds, *La transicion dificil: la autodeterminacion de los pequenos paises perifericos*, Managua: Vanguardia, 1987.
see also: Fagen R, Deere CD, Coraggio JL, eds, *Transition and development: problems of third world socialism*, New York: Monthly Review Press, 1986.
5 Manga P, 'The transformation of Zimbabwe's health care system: a review of the white paper on health', *Social Science and Medicine* 1988; 27(11): 1131-8.
see also: Sanders D, Davies R, 'The economy, the health sector and child health in Zimbabwe since independence', *Social Science and Medicine* 1988; 27(7): 723-31.
6 'The philosophies and policies of the Government of Nicaragua', In: Rosset P, Vandermeer J, eds, *The Nicaragua reader*, New York: Grove Press, 1983.
For material on international health see:
Bryant J, *Health and the developing world*, Ithaca: Cornell University Press, 1969.
Bryant JH, 'Health for all: the dream and the reality', *World Health Forum* 1988; 9: 291-309.
Roemer MI, *National strategies for health care organization*, Ann Arbor: Health Administration Press, 1985.
Roemer MI, 'The changeability of health care systems', *Medical Care* 1986; 24:(1): 24-9.
Roemer MI, *Medical care in Latin America*, Washington, DC: OAS, 1963.
Sidel VW, Sidel R, *A healthy state: an international perspective on the crisis in United States medical care*, New York: Pantheon Books, 1977.
Navarro V, *Medicine under capitalism*, New York: Prodist, 1976.
Basch PF, *Textbook of international health*, New York: Oxford, 1989
7 Direccion Nacional de Atencion Medica, *Atencion primaria de salud en Nicaragua: evolucion historica, logros, y dificultades*, Managua: MINSA, 1984.
see also: Habicht J, Berman PA, 'Strategies in primary health care', *American Journal of Public Health* 1987; 77(11): 1396-7.
8 Navarro V, *Social security and medicine in the USSR: a Marxist critique*, Lexington: Lexington Books, 1977.
9 Harrison P, 'Cuba and Costa Rica: lessons for the third world', *People* 1980; 7(2): 2-4.
10 Nakajima H, 'Health for all: the way ahead', *World Health Forum* 1988; 9: 287-9.

11 Strelnick H, 'Health care under fire: an interview with Dr. Myrna Cunningham', *Health/PAC Bulletin* 1986; 17(1): 15-17.
12 Editorial, *Boletin Cientifico Contingente Medico-Cuban* 1987; 9(2): 1.
13 Halstead SB, Walsh JA, Warren KS, eds, *Good health at low cost*, New York: The Rockefeller Foundation, 1985.
see also: Kendall C, 'The implementation of a diarrhoeal disease control program in Honduras: is it "selective primary health care" or "integrated primary health care"?', *Social Science and Medicine* 1988; 27(1): 17-23.
Smith DL, Bryant JH, 'Building the infrastructure for primary health care: an overview of vertical and integrated approaches', *Social Science and Medicine* 1988; 26(9): 909-17.
Walsh JA, Warren KS, eds, *Strategies for primary health care: technologies appropriate for the control of disease in the developing world*, Chicago: University of Chicago Press, 1986.
14 Grant J, 'The impact of world recession on children', In: Grant J, *The state of the world's children 1988*, New York: Oxford University Press, 1988.
15 Smith DL, Bryant JH, *op. cit.*
16 Ugalde A, 'The role of the medical profession in public health policy making: the case of Colombia', *Social Science and Medicine* 1979; 13(C): 109-19.
17 McMichael JK, ed, *Health in the third world: studies from Vietnam*, Nottingham: Spokesman Books, 1976.

The following references from the international literature on health in Nicaragua are also of interest:

Beson JL, Burges WR, Hull HA, 'Vision care in Nicaragua', *Journal of the American Optometry Association* 1977; 48(8): 1047-51.
Lefton D, 'Nicaragua: health care under the Sandinistas', *Canadian Medical Association Journal* 1984; 130: 781-4.
Lewis V, 'Power or poverty: the riddle of disabled life in Nicaragua', *The Independent* 1980; Fall: 8-29.
Missoni E, Morelli R, 'Survey of 259 cases of American cutaneous leishmaniasis in Nicaragua', *Journal of Tropical Medicine and Hygiene* 1984; 87: 159-65.
Rojas AY, 'Perspectives in international neurosurgery: neurosurgery in Nicaragua', *Neurosurgery* 1980; 7(3): 297-99.
Rosenbaum HD, 'Lessons learned from a radiologic paramedic training effort in Nicaragua', *Diagnostic Imaging* 1982; 51: 180-2.
Sandiford P, Gorter AC, Davey-Smith G, Pauw JPC, 'Determinants of drinking water quality in rural Nicaragua', *Epidemiology and Infection* 1989; 102(2).
Saraceno B, 'L'esperienza psichiatrica in Nicaragua', *The Practioner Edizione Italiana* 1984; 74: 139-45.
Saraceno B, Asioli F, Tognoni G, Flores M, Aguilar R, Sequeira S, *Manual de salud mental (guia basica para atencion primaria)*, Managua: MINSA, 1987.
Tognoni G, 'L'esperanza sanitaria del Nicaragua', *The Practioner Edizione Italiana* 1984; 74: 40-54.

Appendices

Appendix 1: General Health and Economic Data

*Key: * Data Estimated*
- Data Unavailable

	1974	1975	1976	1977	1978	1979	1980	1981	1982	1983	1984	1985	1986	1987	1988	1989
1. Population (000s):																
Total:	2200	2282	2367	2456	2545	2638	2750	2838	2942	3052	3166	3281	3445	3612	3779	3907
Rural:	1100	1141	1160	1180	1222	1240	1286	1305	1324	1343	1361	1378	1396	1414	1431	1463
Towns:	374	365	379	393	407	422	424	426	441	458	475	492	526	558	575	600
Cities:	726	776	828	883	916	976	1040	1107	1177	1251	1330	1411	1523	1640	1771	1844
2. Population Under Five Years Old (000s):	374	388	402	418	433	448	481	511	544	565	586	591	620	632	661	
3. Coverage of Vital Events (%):																
Births:							80	82	80	77	73	68	88	-	-	
Deaths:							42	32	30	41	38	32	47	-	-	
4. Real Salary Relative to 1980:						1.04	1.00	.91	.81	.70	.68	.52	.19			
5. Rate of Inflation (%):						48	35	24	25	31	35	219	682	1200	2000	
6. Per Capita National Product in 1986 Dollars:																
Nicaragua:					1415	1049	1065	1087	1043	1055	1004	931	891	852	758	
Rest of Central America:					1325	1454	1419	1360	1266	1227	1225	1201	1189	1195	1199	
7. Source of MINSA Funds (%):																
Social Security:					65	48	30	26	29	28	26	20	19			
National Lottery*:					3	3	4	4	4	4	4	4	4			
Central Government:					32	49	67	51	51	56	65	77	78			

	1974	1975	1976	1977	1978	1979	1980	1981	1982	1983	1984	1985	1986	1987	1988	1989
8. Health as % of Gross Domestic Production:					1.8	2.5	3.2	4.7	4.9	4.7	4.8	6.0	7.0	7.8		
9. Proportion of National Budget to (%):																
Health:					8	10	11	13	11	9	7	9	11	9		
Other Social:							15	16	14	13	13	14	15	15		
Defence:							20	22	19	20	23	35	38	46		
Production:							52	49	56	58	57	42	36	30		
10. MINSA Foreign Expenditure in Millions of Dollars:																
Dollars Spent:							46	64	48	58	29	55	41	23		
MINSA Debt:							0	0	0	11	15	20	18	18		
Donations Received:							12	13	6	21	12	9	6	8		
11. Doctors:	928	911	1131	1319	1492	1345	1349	1445	1626	1802	1880	1786	1814	1471		
12. Nurses:	379	395	442	566	379	640	808	900	795	1182	1271	1046	1158	1267		
13. Dentists:	72	86	96	139	153	179	190	183	191	222	222	260	305	263		
14. Auxiliary Nurses:	1870	2120	2261	2940	1873	3176	3879	3884	3995	4226	4378	4126	4421	5296		
15. New Graduate Doctors:	*50	*50	*50	*50	60	72	80	172	121	117	213	341	274	261		
16. New Graduate Nurses:	79	56	76	73	106	136	150	197	110	162	192	177	125	279		

	1974	1975	1976	1977	1978	1979	1980	1981	1982	1983	1984	1985	1986	1987	1988	1989
17. New Graduate Auxiliary Nurses:	103	128	131	54	167	230	603	738	574	338	234	321	452	586		
18. Total MINSA Labour Force (00s):							158	154	179	208	216	223	232	213		
19. Left MINSA Labour Force (00s):							-	-	-	23	56	60	74	45		
20. Health Workers Mobilised to the Army (00s):								51	71	157	196	153	-	-		
21. Regional Variation in Health Personnel per 10,000 Population:																
Region With Highest Rate of Doctors:							9.0	7.9	8.2	9.3	10.6	9.6	8.6	9.1	8.0	
Region With Lowest Rate of Doctors:							1.4	1.9	3.0	4.1	4.0	3.6	2.6	2.0	3.5	
Region With Highest Rate of Nurses:							3.4	5.2	4.6	3.5	6.6	5.7	3.7	4.3	4.5	
Region With Lowest Rate of Nurses:							0.1	1.2	1.8	1.9	2.5	2.6	1.8	2.3	2.2	
Region With Highest Rate of Auxiliary Nurses:							12.4	19.3	17.2	17.0	19.3	16.6	16.1	13.7	13.9	
Region With Lowest Rate of Auxiliary Nurses:							1.4	7.8	8.6	7.6	6.0	7.0	8.9	7.8	7.3	
22. Prescriptions Dispensed (0000s):	575	560	726	778	680	788	896	1039	1161	1303	1458	1545	1439	1338		
23. Laboratory Examinations (00s):	1420	1539	1929	2452	2351	-	3046	3133	3625	3822	3741	3617	3846	3869		
24. X-Rays (00s):	1370	1680	2100	2590	2350	2270	3090	3370	4050	3940	3640	3290	3657	3634		
25. Beds in Public Hospitals:	3991	4115	4272	4313	4409	4000	4677	4729	4765	4897	5045	5010	4925	4898		

	1974	1975	1976	1977	1978	1979	1980	1981	1982	1983	1984	1985	1986	1987	1988	1989
26. Hospitalisations (000s):	107	108	121	125	136	155	178	191	197	207	200	202	215	223		
27. Surgical Procedures (00s):	24	28	35	36	25	-	54	54	56	54	56	56	61	66		
28. Dental Visits (00s):	1240	1530	1770	2040	1790	1100	2590	3320	4170	4400	4290	4600	5230	5599		
29. Births in Health Institutions (00s):	320	350	360	419	400	-	516	556	580	607	582	579	654	591		
30. Medical Visits (000s):	1837	1939	1953	2433	1769	2117	4982	5411	6034	6334	6045	5654	6150	6460		
31. Medical Visits at (000s):																
Clinics and Health Posts:							3025	3122	3825	4273	3799	3609	4479	4913		
Hospitals:							1925	2289	2209	2061	2246	2045	1671	1547		
32. Per Capita Medical Visits:																
Region 1:				0.2	-	-	1.4	1.7	2.1	2.4	2.1	1.9	1.9	1.7		
Region 2:				0.9	-	-	1.5	1.4	1.6	1.9	1.7	1.7	1.8	1.8		
Region 3:				2.1	-	-	2.8	2.9	2.6	3.0	2.3	2.2	2.0	2.1		
Region 4:				0.5	-	-	1.7	1.8	1.9	2.0	1.8	1.3	1.6	1.7		
Region 5:				0.2	-	-	1.4	1.1	1.4	1.2	1.3	1.2	1.4	1.8		
Region 6:				0.3	-	-	0.7	1.3	1.8	1.6	1.8	1.8	1.9	1.8		
Autonomous Zone:				0.9	-	-	2.2	2.4	2.9	2.0	2.2	2.0	2.2	1.8		

	1974	1975	1976	1977	1978	1979	1980	1981	1982	1983	1984	1985	1986	1987	1988	1989
33. Per Capita Medical Visits by Age, National:																
Under One-Year-Olds:										3.8	3.2	2.4	4.4	4.6		
Age 1 to 4 years:										1.6	1.5	1.0	1.8	1.8		
Age 5 to 14 years:										0.9	0.8	0.8	0.9	0.9		
Over Age 15:										1.5	1.4	1.3	2.0	2.1		
34. Per Capita Medical Visits by Age, Managua:																
Under One-Year-Olds:										7.0	-	4.0	-	3.8		
Age 1 to 4 years :										2.9	-	1.8	-	1.5		
Age 5 to 14 years:										1.1	-	0.8	-	0.7		
Over Age 15:										3.7	-	2.7	-	2.8		
35. Visits for Nutritional Monitoring (000s):								176	314	382	438	433	493	542		
36. Well-Child Visits (000s):								128	287	438	403	429	495	467		
37. Visits for Prenatal Care (000s):								138	245	303	318	316	360	383		
38. Visits for Birth Control (000s):																
Total:								24	81	142	137	201	264	292		
Pills:								15	60	106	104	161	222	234		
IUDs:								2	8	15	17	21	24	27		
Other:								6	13	22	16	20	19	25		
39. Visits for Puerperal Care (000s):								7	25	43	43	47	60	61		
40. Visits for Pap Smears (000s):								-	-	22	26	41	54	62		

	1974	1975	1976	1977	1978	1979	1980	1981	1982	1983	1984	1985	1986	1987	1988	1989
41. Gastroenteritis Treatments Among:																
Hospital Inpatients (000s):							14	15	15	17	15	15	15	15		
Hospital Outpatients (000s):							42	52	67	76	79	99	99	81		
Health Centres (000s):							157	191	237	265	266	257	266	243		
Oral Rehydration Centres (000s):							72	96	141	172	173	202	248	264		
42. Gastroenteritis Treatments in Oral Rehydration Centres:																
Referred for IV Treatment (000s):							2	2	3	3	2	3	3	3		
Oral Treatment, Referred to Home (000s):							29	42	60	90	99	103	101	101		
Oral Treatment, at URO (000s):							40	52	77	78	71	96	144	159		
43. Health Volunteers Trained (000s):								-	20	21	20	14	11	-		
44. Health Centres Without Beds:	92	116	127	152	163	146	88	89	85	87	86	83	76	82		
45. Health Centres With Beds:	1	1	1	1	1	1	11	15	13	17	18	22	24	23		
46. Health Posts:	38	0	0	19	25	25	267	358	354	348	323	281	249	348		
47. War-Affected Health Posts:							0	0	8	36	59	82	102	119		
48. Hospitals Inaugurated:						0	0	1	0	3	0	1	1	0		
49. Amputations Performed, By Reasons:																
Mines and Explosives:						13	3	5	6	10	23	28	20	132	50	
Other:						7	4	11	6	5	10	17	109	79	15	

	1974	1975	1976	1977	1978	1979	1980	1981	1982	1983	1984	1985	1986	1987	1988	1989
50. Number of People Displaced by Contra War (000s):										91	143	120	97	81		
51. Number of Casualties Among Health Workers:																
Wounded:							0	0	0	5	2	5	4	9		
Kidnapped:							0	3	0	4	10	11	1	2		
Killed:							1	1	3	13	11	11	2	3		
52. Number of Casualties Among General Population:																
Wounded:								26	156	1157	561	790	1852	3763		
Kidnapped:								23	306	530	645	832	1455	2846		
Killed:								66	500	646	1099	1341	347	1715		
53. Reported Cases of Whooping Cough:	2219	1390	853	791	623	267	2469	1935	395	97	60	150	223	293		
54. Reported Cases of Measles:	853	1765	1361	901	161	1270	3784	224	226	112	153	956	2021	794		
55. Reported Cases of Tetanus:	72	59	13	18	13	-	89	132	115	177	97	76	84	44		
56. Reported Tetanus Deaths:	207	227	229	237	109	-	153	127	109	120	50	42	48			
57. Reported Cases of Malaria (00s):	122	247	262	116	106	184	255	174	156	129	157	151	170	169		
In Non-war Zone:									91	26	35	32	40	31		
In War Zone:									65	103	122	119	130	138		

	1974	1975	1976	1977	1978	1979	1980	1981	1982	1983	1984	1985	1986	1987	1988	1989
58. Reported Cases of Polio:																
	43	40	1	36	1	101	21	45	0	0	0	0	0	0		
59. Measles Vaccine Doses Administered by:																
Volunteers (000s):								132	125	153	175	130	108	78		
Health System (000s):				92	-	-	102	96	80	81	98	157	142	114		
60. Polio Vaccine Doses Administered by:																
Volunteers (000s):								642	1123	1343	1643	1649	1708	1256		
Health System (000s):	233	757	504	643	384	-	538	521	367	473	429	540	552	499		
61. Coverage Among Children Under One Year of Age with Vaccines Against (%):																
Tuberculosis:					24	-	33	65	82	88	98	99	69	94		
Polio:					17	-	21	24	70	82	77	84	94	85		
Diptheria, Tetanus, Pertusis:					18	-	15	23	26	24	33	42	45	56		
Measles:					-	-	15	20	40	41	56	59	51	45		
62. Numbers of Children Served By Social Welfare Centres (0s):																
Urban Food Centres:								178	179	121	170	200	230	440		
Rural Food Centres:								150	395	487	1000	1400	1650	1913		
Urban Child Care:							62	163	206	294	300	330	354	412		
Rural Child Care:								67	187	267	190	290	390	446		
63. Estimated Infant Mortality Rate (per 1000 Live Births):																
National:	99	97	94	92	90	89	85	81	77	73	72	70	68	68		
Rural:	105	103	100	97	95	92	89	86	83	80	78	76	74	74		
Urban:	82	81	79	78	77	76	75	73	71	70	68	66	64	64		

	1974	1975	1976	1977	1978	1979	1980	1981	1982	1983	1984	1985	1986	1987	1988	1989
64. Value of Agricultural Exports in Millions of Current Dollars:																
Coffee:										153	118	107	115	88		
Cotton:										110	91	41	43	50		
Beef:										31	11	5	13	20		
Sugar:										34	7	9	8	5		
Bananas:										15	16	14	15	-		
65. Per Capita Food Availability:																
Eggs (Dozens):				5.3	-	-	-	11.7	-	-	12.8	-				
Oil (Litres):				19.4	-	-	-	22.9	-	-	22.9	-				
Meat (Pounds):				26.5	-	-	-	32.1	-	-	29.9	-				
Beans (Pounds):				38.6	-	-	-	38.1	-	-	45.1	-				
Rice (Pounds):				45.2	-	-	-	55.1	-	-	76.1	-				
Sugar (Pounds):				103.9	-	-	-	91.1	-	-	101.1	-				
Maize (Pounds):				174.4	-	-	-	173.9	-	-	152.1	-				
66. Percent of Population with Access to Piped Water:																
Urban:	72	-	-	-	-	63	-	-	-	-	-	76				
Rural:	6	-	-	-	-	6	-	-	-	-	-	11				
67. Metric Tons of Food Imported:																
Maize:	1	10	46	11	38	3	114	73	54	300	176	337	171			
Beans:	7	3	.2	.2	2	2	27	58	4	6	10	12	5			
68. Metric Tons of Food Produced:																
Maize:	415	414	417	437	394	552	375	399	419	400	508	467	514	530		
Beans:	74	101	96	117	89	120	86	62	90	103	138	128	119	148		
Rice:	112	146	122	82	105	130	93	139	202	214	212	194	226	246		

69. Per Capita Health Spending By Region in Current *Cordobas*:

	1972	**1986**
National Average:	43	6925
Region 1:	16	4404
Region 2:	134	5825
Region 3:	228	9259
Region 4:	50	4797
Region 5:	2	4447
Region 6:	20	3419
Autonomous Zone:	40	8866

70. Infant Deaths per 10,000 Births 1985/86:

	Vaccine-Preventable Infections	Respiratory	Gastroenteritis	Perinatal	Other
Nicaragua:	5	84	228	256	99
Honduras:	82	143	308	157	120

71. Deaths per 10,000 Children Aged One to Four Years Old:

	Vaccine-Preventable Infections	Respiratory	Gastroenteritis	Violence	Other Infections	Other
1975/76	6	18	48	6	14	16
1985/86	10	15	22	10	8	21

72. Infant Mortality Rate by Mother's Education:

	No School		Primary	Secondary
1966/67	136		108	57
1973/74	112		91	47
	Illiterate	Literate		
1982/83	91	73	71	46

73. Reported and Estimated Rate of Death per 1000 Population, By Age, 1986:

Age:	Deaths Registered In Hospitals	Total Deaths Registered	Total Estimated Number of Deaths
Under One Year:	16	31	55
1-4 Years:	1	1.5	9
5-14 Years:	0.2	0.5	2
15-49 Years:	0.5	2.1	3
50 Years or More:	4	16	27

74. Percent of all Health Personnel Working in Primary Care:

	1971	1981	1986
Nurses:	11	30	28
Doctors:	12	36	30
Auxiliary Nurses:	9	30	47

75. Percent of Under-Five-Year-Olds Malnourished:

	Moderate	Severe
1966	29	17
1977	35	19
1981	33	17
1988	31	16

Appendix 2
Comparative Data on Health and Social Conditions in Central America
(1984 or 1985 unless otherwise stated)

	Nicaragua	Honduras	Costa Rica	El Salvador	Guatemala
76. Population in Millions:	3.2	4.3	2.6	5.5	7.9
77. % Rural:	43	60	52	47	62
78. GNP per Capita in Current Dollars:	880	670	1670	680	1110
79. Last Year in Which Real Per Capita Income Was as Low As 1985:	1962	1971	1975	1965	1974
80. % Value of Currency Compared With 1979 Value:	3	53	16	37	38
81. Literacy Rate 1980/1985:	88/85	67/59	90/94	57/72	57/55
82. Infant Mortality Rate/1000	72	82	20	71	68
83. Life Expectancy At Birth:	60	60	73	65	59
84. Population per Doctor:	1800	3120	1460	3220	8610
85. Rate of Population Growth:	3.4	3.4	2.7	3.0	2.9
86. % of Population Indigenous:	2	3	1	2	60

	Nicaragua	Honduras	Costa Rica	El Salvador	Guatemala
87. Population per Square Km.:	24	39	51	265	73
88. Public Spending as % of GNP:	58	25	18	21	11
89. % Population Poor and Very Poor in 1980:	62	68	25	68	71
90. % Population Very Poor in 1980:	35	57	14	50	40
91. % of National Income Going to Poorest 40% of Population Around 1975:	9	7	12	16	13
92. % of National Income Going to Richest 20% of Population Around 1975:	65	68	55	47	60
93. % of Urban Population With Adequate Water Access in 1979:	81	92	100	67	89
94. % of Urban Population With Toilets in 1979:	31	43	43	47	34
95. % of Children Fully Immunised Against Polio at Age 1:	70	58	75	54	21

	Nicaragua	Honduras	Costa Rica	El Salvador	Guatemala
96. % of Births Medically Assisted:	38	34	96	34	16
97. Population Age Structure:					
0-9	34	34	26	32	33
10-19	24	24	21	25	23
20-64	40	39	49	39	41
65+	3	3	4	3	3

Appendix 3

98. Number and Rank of Principal Causes of Death Among Hospitalised Patients, 1980 - 1986

Diagnosis	1980	1981	1982	1983	1984	1985	1986
Intestinal Infections:	510(1)	291(3)	216(6)	331(4)	286(6)	325(5)	411(5)
Pneumonia:	498(2)	281(4)	220(5)	342(3)	292(5)	304(6)	429(4)
Septicaemia:	434(3)	321(1)	333(2)	385(2)	330(4)	366(4)	253(7)
Late Foetal Growth and Malnutrition:	292(4)	300(2)	399(1)	306(6)	262(7)	275(7)	277(6)
Perinatal Causes:	266(5)	257(5)	227(4)	318(5)	375(2)	451(2)	447(2)
Hypoxia and Other Neonatal Causes:	214(6)	257(6)	283(3)	401(1)	440(1)	373(3)	435(3)
Poorly Defined Causes:	146(7)	178(7)	213(7)	272(7)	331(3)	468(1)	(1)

( ) *Indicates Rank As Cause of Death in Hospitals*

Appendix 4

99. Demographic Variables, 1950 - 1985

	1950-55	55-60	60-65	65-70	70-75	75-80	80-85
Total Fertility Rate: *(Average Number of Total Children per Woman)*	7.3	7.3	7.3	7.1	6.7	6.3	5.9
Crude Birth Rate: *(Births per 1000 inhabitants)*	54	52	50	48	47	46	44
Crude Death Rate: *(Deaths per 1000 inhabitants)*	23	20	17	15	13	12	10
Population Growth Rate: *(Percent annual increase in the population)*	3.1	3.2	3.2	3.2	3.2	2.8	3.4
Life Expectancy at Birth: *(In Years)*	42	45	49	52	55	56	60

Appendix 5

100. Age Specific Hospital Admission and Mortality Rates for Diarrhoeal Diseases, 1980 - 1986

Age at Admission	**Years**						
	1980	**1981**	**1982**	**1983**	**1984**	**1985**	**1986**
1 - 27 days:	964 (6.7)	757 (6.5)	944 (3.3)	961 (4.3)	859 (4.1)	689 (3.5)	758 (5.9)
28 days - 11 months:	9013 (3.6)	9271 (1.9)	9514 (1.6)	11347 (1.9)	10065 (2.1)	8702 (2.7)	7969 (3.7)
1 - 4 years:	2904 (3.6)	3079 (1.9)	3362 (0.7)	3284 (1.5)	2926 (1.1)	2441 (2.0)	2103 (2.4)
5 - 14 years:	453 (3.8)	433 (1.6)	380 (0.8)	380 (1.3)	304 (1.3)	304 (1.0)	266 (1.5)
15 - 49 years:	762 (0.4)	737 (0.4)	680 (0.1)	710 (1.5)	613 (0.5)	641 (0.5)	528 (0.8)
50+ years:	323 (1.9)	362 (1.9)	355 (2.3)	415 (3.9)	488 (2.5)	468 (1.7)	467 (2.7)
Total:	**14419 (3.6)**	**14639 (2.1)**	**15235 (1.5)**	**17097 (2.0)**	**15255 (2.0)**	**13245 (2.5)**	**12091 (3.4)**

( ) *Indicates Mortality Rate*

Appendix 6

101. Total Number of Deaths Recorded, by Cause, 1983 - 1986

Diagnosis	1983	1984	1985	1986
Intestinal Infections:	1523	1425	1386	1714
Pulmonary Diseases and Other Heart Diseases:	979	843	1008	705
Pneumonia:	820	1000	304	696
Malignant Tumours:	474	731	813	1617
Cerebrovascular Diseases:	748	718	825	805
Late Foetal Development, Malnutrition, and Prematurity:	464	621	696	707

Appendix 7: References for the Appendices

1 and 2. Official population estimates for Nicaragua are provided by INEC via demographic projections based on the 1971 national census. This was the last reliable census carried out throughout the country. These are sometimes adjusted on the basis of special surveys or revised demographic assumptions. The data presented here represent slightly higher population estimates, based in part on the following sources:
Republica de Nicaragua, *Censos nacionales 1971*, Managua: Gobierno de Nicaragua, 1974.
BCN, *Compendio estadistico 1965 - 1974*, Managua: BCN, 1975.
CEPAL, *Anuario estadistico de America Latina*, Chile: CEPAL, 1984.
IADB, *Report on demographic trends and projections for Central America*, Washington, DC: IADB, 1977.
Fox RW, Huguet JW, *Population and urban trends in Central America and Panama*, Washington DC: IADB, 1977.

3. INEC. Derived by comparing data on registered events to demographic projections of expected number of births and deaths.
4. Derived by comparing mid-year black market exchange rates with the US dollar to average *cordoba* salary levels. 1988 data from Uhlig M, 'Nicaraguan study depicts economy in drastic decline', *New York Times*, 1/26/89, p.1.
5. Ministerio de Finanza.
6. Interamerican Development Bank.
7. Direccion de Finanza, MINSA and INSSBI.
8. Ministerio de Finanza and Direccion de Finanza, MINSA.
9. Ministerio de Finanza.
10. MINSA, *Plan de salud 1988 - 1990*, Managua: MINSA 1987.
11. DINEI.
12. DINEI.
13. DINEI.
14. DINEI.
15. DINEI.
16. DINEI.
17. DINEI.
18. MINSA, *Plan de salud 1988 - 1990*, Managua: MINSA 1987.
19. MINSA, *Plan de salud 1988 - 1990*, Managua: MINSA 1987.
20. CONAPRO Heroes y Martires, and MINSA, Oficina de Defensa Civil.
21. DINEI.
22. DINEI.
23. DINEI.
24. DINEI.
25. DINEI.
26. DINEI.
27. DINEI.
28. DINEI.
29. DINEI.

30. DINEI.
31. DINEI.
32. DINEI.
33. MINSA, *Plan de salud 1988 - 1990*, Managua: MINSA 1987.
34. MINSA Region 3, *Plan de Salud 1988*, Managua: MINSA, 1988.
35. DINEI.
36. DINEI.
37. DINEI.
38. DINEI.
39. DINEI.
40. DINEI.
41. DINEI.
42. DINEI.
43. DECOPS.
44. DINEI.
45. DINEI.
46. DINEI.
47. MINSA, Oficina de Defensa Civil.
48. MINSA, *Plan de salud 1988 - 1990*, Managua: MINSA 1987.
49. CARE, *Children's survival assistance programme needs assessment team field report: Nicaragua*, New York: CARE, 1988.
50. INSSBI.
51. MINSA, Oficina de Defensa Civil.
52. Secretaria de la Junta de Gobierno.
53. Direccion de Epidemiologia, MINSA.
54. Direccion de Epidemiologia, MINSA.
55. Direccion de Epidemiologia, MINSA.
56. Direccion de Epidemiologia, MINSA.
57. Direccion de Epidemiologia, MINSA.
58. Direccion de Epidemiologia, MINSA.
59. DINEI.
60. DINEI.
61. PAHO, *Health conditions in the Americas 1981 - 1984*, Washington, DC: PAHO, 1986 and
    PAHO, *Health conditions in the Americas 1977-1980*, Washington, DC: PAHO, 1982.
62. INSSBI.
63. Although estimates vary widely on national infant mortality levels in Nicaragua and other Central American countries, an extensive review carried out by Dr. Hugo Behm in 1987 provides the most reliable estimates available. Estimates were included only for years with data points in the figure. Data for intervening years were extrapolated from those years for which there were data points. Limitations of the data and a discussion of the primary studies included are provided in:
    CELADE, *La mortalidad en la ninez en Centroamerica, Panama and Belice: Nicaragua 1970-1986*, San Jose: CELADE, 1988.
64. *Barricada Internacional*, 12/8/88, p.3 and Corporacion Nicaraguense de Empresas de Comercio Exterior, *Boletin Informativo 1988;* 10/11.
65. Fitzgerald V, 'Agrarian reform as a model of accumulation: the case of

Nicaragua since 1979', *Journal of Development Studies* 1985; 22:1.
66. CIERA, Informe de Nicaragua a la FAO, Managua: CIERA, 1983.
MINSA, *Analisis preliminar de la situation de salud en Nicaragua. Tomo II: unidad de analisis del sector salud*, 1979.
MINSA, *Plan de salud 1988 - 1990*, Managua: MINSA 1987.
67. Zalkin M, 'Food policy and class transformation in revolutionary Nicaragua, 1979 - 86', *World Development* 1987; 15 (7): 961 - 84 and
Banco Central de Nicaragua.
68. Zalkin M. *op. cit.*
69. MINSA, *Analisis preliminar de la situation de salud en Nicaragua. Tomo II: unidad de analisis del sector salud*, 1979 and MINSA, Plan de salud 1987, Managua: MINSA, 1986.
70. CELADE, *La mortalidad en la ninez en Centroamerica, Panama and Belice: Nicaragua 1970-1986*, San Jose: CELADE, 1988.
71. *ibid.*
72. *ibid.*
73. DINEI and INEC.
74. DINEI and Bartlett L, 'Nicaragua health services referral system: a preliminary report', unpublished 1976.
76. CEPAL, *Anuario estadistico de America Latina*, Chile: CEPAL, 1984.
77. *ibid.*
78. Westinghouse Corporation, *Child survival, risks, and the road to health*, Columbia MD: Institute for Research Development, 1987.
79. Gallardo ME, Lopez JR, *Centro America: la crisis en cifras*, Costa Rica: Flasco, 1986.
80. CEPAL, *Informe anual sobre America Latina*, Mexico: CEPAL, 1986.
IADB, *Economic and social progress in Latin America*, Washington, DC: IADB, 1983.
81. Grant J, *State of the world's children report, 1989*, New York: Oxford University Press, 1988.
82. *ibid.*
83. *ibid.*
84. CEPAL, *Anuario estadistico de America Latina*, Chile: CEPAL, 1984.
85. *ibid.*
86. Wilkie I, Peokel A, eds, *Statistical abstract of Latin America*, Los Angeles: University of California Press, 1986.
87. CEPAL, *Anuario estadistico de America Latina*, Chile: CEPAL, 1984.
88. Consejo Monetario Centroamericano, *Boletin estadistico*, Costa Rica: Consejo Monetario Centroamericano, 1984.
89. CEPAL, *Notas sobre la evolucion del desarollo social del Istmo Centroamericana hasta 1980*, Mexico: CEPAL, 1980.
90. *ibid.*
91. *ibid.*
92. *ibid.*
93. CEPAL, *Anuario estadistico de America Latina*, Chile: CEPAL, 1984.
94. *ibid.*
95. PAHO, *Health conditions in the Americas 1981 - 1984*, Washington, DC: PAHO, 1986
96 *ibid.*

97. UNESCO, *Apoyo a acciones estrategicos de escolarizacion, alfabetizacion, y mejoramiento de la calidad de la educacion en Centroamerica Y Panama*, Costa Rica: UNESCO 514/RLA/11, 1988.
98. DINEI.
99. Oficina Ejecutiva de Encuestas y Censos, '25 anos de estadistica vital', *Boletin Demografico* 1978; 3.
100. DINEI.
101. INEC.

THE NICARAGUA HEALTH FUND

The Nicaragua Health Fund works in partnership with Nicaragua's health workers supporting their pioneering primary health programmes and helping to maintain hospital services. Founded in 1986 the work of the Health Fund has grown rapidly to encompass a wide range of programmes including:

Working in the war zones: Boaco and Chontales are remote and underdeveloped regions in which the difficult task of providing health care to a scattered population has been made worse by almost a decade of Contra attacks and compounded by the destruction caused by Hurricane Joan in October 1988. Here NHF has funded a number of projects including the training of traditional midwives and health brigadistas and the construction of two rural health posts. This area of particular need will continue to be a priority for NHF for the foreseeable future.

Child to child: In Nicaragua over half the population is under 15. In such a young country it is often the older children rather than their parents who care for their younger brothers and sisters. With this in mind, NHF is supporting an exciting new project in which 9-12 year olds are taught the basics of preventative medicine and primary health care. Through songs, games and role-plays they learn to spot the early signs of illness and disability in their siblings and playmates and how to prevent common diseases.

Sending a lifeline: "We have to re-use disposable syringes so often you can hear the skin break" (British health worker in Nicaragua). Hospital services in Nicaragua are in crisis. Shortages of the most basic supplies hamper every aspect of their work. Since 1987 NHF has been sending over containers of medical goods to supplement the country's supplies. In 1988 alone £173,000 worth of supplies were collected from hospitals and manufacturers by volunteers. As the economic crisis deepens this lifeline becomes ever more vital.

Making the links: As well as having an important role to play in supporting health work in Nicaragua through material and financial aid, we in Britain also have much to learn from Nicaragua's creative new approach to health care. NHF works to increase awareness of the current situation, the needs and the lessons through a regular newsletter, publications, study tours, exhibitions and conferences.

This work is all made possible by the generous contributions of individual supporters. Anyone wishing to find out more, make a donation or join the Nicaragua Health Fund should write to:

Nicaragua Health Fund, 83 Margaret Street, London W1N 7HB. Tel. 01 580 4292.

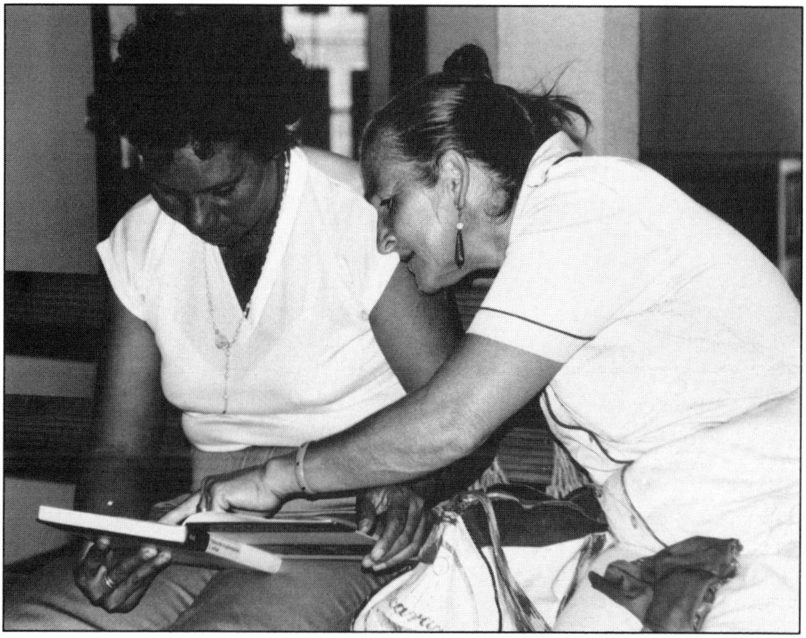

Traditional midwives are now recognised as valuable contributors to health teams. NHF is paying for their training in Boaco and Chontales.